Dr. Heimlich's Home Guide to

Emergency Medical Situations

by Henry J. Heimlich, M.D., with Lawrence Galton

A FIRESIDE BOOK
Published by Simon & Schuster, Inc.
NEW YORK

Copyright © 1980 by Henry J. Heimlich, M.D.,
and Lawrence Galton
First Fireside Edition, 1984
Published by Simon & Schuster, Inc.
Simon & Schuster Building
Rockefeller Center
1230 Avenue of the Americas
New York, New York 10020

FIRESIDE and colophon are registered trademarks
of Simon & Schuster, Inc.

Designed by Irving Perkins

Manufactured in the United States of America

10 9 8 7 6 5 4 3 2
10 9 8 7 6 5 4 3 2 1 Pbk.

Library of Congress Cataloging in Publication Data

Heimlich, Henry J
Dr. Heimlich's Home Guide to Emergency Medical
Situations.

    Includes index.
    1. Medical emergencies. 2. First aid in illness and injury.
I. Galton, Lawrence, joint author.
II. Title
RC86.7.H42   616'.025   79-21638

ISBN 0-671-24947-9
ISBN 0-671-53075-5 Pbk.

Contents

Introduction:
A Personal Word
to the Reader

Behind this book lie a story and a concept. The concept has to do with the medical emergencies in your life—*all* the situations that really, and rightly, fall into the emergency category.

The story has to do with a tragic incident.

What has come to be known as the *Heimlich maneuver* was first described in June 1974, in a medical journal, *Emergency Medicine*. That same month, the simple huglike maneuver for saving the life of a person choking on food was successfully used by a lay person.

But at about the same time at a medical dinner meeting in Washington, D.C., a physician choked to death on a chunk of food as one hundred other physicians sat helplessly by, not realizing why their colleague had fallen unconscious and was dying.

The diagnosis of choking on food had been left so complex that even a large group of physicians failed to recognize the tragedy occurring in their midst.

Please bear with me for a moment about the story of the maneuver and how it relates to you.

The maneuver was developed after many laboratory studies. They showed that even in the midst of choking and inability to breathe, a substantial amount of air is left

1

in the lungs. And they showed, too, that if you press your fist into a choking person's abdomen and thrust upward on the diaphragm, you compress the lungs and force the remaining air out through the windpipe—with such force that this air literally pops the obstruction out of the throat and mouth.

But if the maneuver were to be useful, recognition of choking had to be simplified so that the diagnosis could be made promptly by anyone—by a nearby diner in a restaurant, a family member at the dinner table at home, a mother whose child comes running because he is choking on a toy—for there are only four minutes to act. In four minutes life is lost.

It became possible, after analyzing what happens during choking, to establish a 1, 2, 3 order of events:

1. The person cannot breathe—*and cannot speak* (because his airway is blocked and no air can pass through the vocal cords).
2. He turns *blue* (because oxygen is not getting to body tissues).
3. He falls unconscious (because oxygen is not getting to his brain).

Then later, happily, the public contributed. As the maneuver became increasingly known, many people wrote. "Since the choking victim cannot speak," they suggested, "why not provide a signal he can use to indicate his condition to others." They suggested waiving a finger, or hitting the top of the head with the flat of a hand, or throwing a plate against a wall.

It was with the help of a school for the deaf that I

devised what is known now as the *Heimlich sign:* hand to neck. When a choking victim spreads a hand over the front of his neck, it says to anyone who has learned the signal (and millions now have): "Help me! I'm choking!" A potential rescuer then need only ask: "Are you choking?" And the victim can nod his head.

Both the 1, 2, 3 breakdown and sign as well as the maneuver have been much publicized through the media and through illustrated wall charts in public eating places and elsewhere.

The result has been a saving of more than 20,000 lives in fifteen years.

Choking on food or another object is only one emergency situation. There are, of course, many more that involve life or death or serious disfigurement and disability—many of them long recognized to be situations requiring quick, knowledgeable treatment. You will find them in the pages that follow. You will also find many other conditions beyond those ordinarily thought of as medical emergencies.

Yes, it is an emergency if you suffer a serious fall, a severe burn, break a limb, are badly bruised or cut. It is also an emergency if you suffer, or think you may be suffering, a heart attack; if you wake up in the middle of the night with a severe bellyache; if you get up in the morning with a stiff and painful neck; if suddenly a crop of hives covers your body. It can be an emergency if suddenly you develop severe itching, an outbreak of boils, a crop of painful canker sores, a headache that follows a seemingly minor head injury a few days before and refuses to vanish.

What this book tries to do is to break down such

conditions to their basics: to make it easier for you to recognize what may be wrong; to guide you, whenever possible, to treating it successfully yourself; and to guide you, too, to recognizing when you really do need medical help—and how soon.

I think you may find, too, that in those situations where you do need medical or surgical help, you will benefit by a greater understanding of what goes into the physician's diagnosis and what goes into effective treatment.

I hope you will find that what was planned for this book—to make it complete, direct and practical, with a format to enable you to find what you need quickly*—is realized and valuable to you. This guide clearly is intended for use in emergencies when there is not time to obtain trained professional advice and help.

I think you will find the "Read This Now" pages that immediately follow especially valuable. And I urge you to read them first.

HENRY J. HEIMLICH, M.D.

*Entries are arranged alphabetically and cross-referenced where necessary.

NOTE: *This is not a substitute for seeking medical attention, and we cannot be responsible for misinterpretation or misuse of recommendations.*

Part One

Read This Now

Why Now

Almost certainly, there are many pages throughout this book to which you will be referring at some time in the future, and some you may have reason to consult now because they may serve an immediate need.

These next pages, however, are indeed special, and I hope very much that you will read them now and perhaps come back to review them at regular intervals.

They are important because they contain information you should know about in advance of emergency—facts, insights, procedures that can help you to act promptly, knowingly, effectively.

They are important, too, because they can help you in some situations to avoid well-meant but misguided, outdated advice and directions from other sources, including some you may, understandably enough, believe to be authentic.

And they are important, some in particular, for attitude of mind.

"Look at the Bleeding" is very much concerned with attitude. I think you will agree that it will be an attitude you will want to transmit to your children to serve them

5

throughout their lives, and enable them to react to emergency situations and illness calmly, with understanding and without panic.

The section on POISONING can help you avoid mistakes—some of them potentially disastrous—that might not be your fault but rather due to outdated first aid labels, now known to be mistaken but still carried on many dangerous household products.

Your understanding of the section on SHOCK—on how to recognize as well as combat it—can make a life and death difference in many accidents and other medical emergency situations. Shock can be a needless killer.

The two sections on ABDOMINAL PAIN and CHEST PAIN will give you insights into their many possible causes and help you determine what is going on and what to do when either of these very common symptoms occurs.

CHOKING . . . AND THE HEIMLICH MANEUVER—here, too, it is essential to know in advance how to recognize the former and how to apply the latter without even a few minutes' delay.

Similarly, the CPR (cardiopulmonary resuscitation) section belongs here because there is little time for you to first read about it when a life is at stake.

The section on BURNS prepares you to quickly size up the seriousness of a burn and, accordingly, what to do promptly for it.

Perhaps at first blush the COUGHING section may seem out of place. Yet coughing is often misunderstood and mistreated. You will find it rewarding to know that there are times when you should not only not suppress but instead *encourage* it—and *HOW* to do that.

I have included here, too, suggestions on how to

stock emergency kits—for your home, for your car, for usual travel, and for travel that may take you beyond medical aid.

"Look at the Bleeding!"

How we react—or how our parents react—when we first cut or injure ourselves and become aware of bleeding can affect our response to injuries and illnesses throughout our lives.

Do consider:

When a child comes running to a parent with a small amount of blood trickling through the skin—or, for that matter, a large amount—if the parent becomes alarmed and panicky, the tension will be transmitted immediately to the child who, for the rest of his or her life, is likely to react with the same alarm and panic at the sight of blood and in the face of other injury or illness.

If parent or child becomes sufficiently upset to faint, the situation is further worsened.

Yet a fairly substantial amount of blood can be lost—in an adult as much as a pint, in a child a little less—with little or no serious effect.

Should anyone in your family suffer an injury that leads to bleeding, simply hold the arm or leg or whatever other part of the body is bleeding, and say quietly: "Well, look at the blood; isn't that great! It washes out the wound so the germs which got in when you cut yourself will not stay in there."

Say to the child: "Do look. It's really a wonderful process. And now that it has done its work, we'll soon stop it."

When that child grows up, he will know how to react

calmly and constructively to emergencies and, as well, to disease.

The first thing to do with any such cut or bruise is to wash it with clear, cold water and advise the child that this may cause a little burning sensation. Explain that the reason for the burning sensation is that the place where the skin is cut or broken has left some nerves exposed— but don't worry; they will heal.

If possible, wash the area surrounding the wound with soap and water. Do not be concerned if, as you rinse the soap off the surrounding area of skin, a little of the soap-containing rinse water washes into the wound; it further cleanses it.

For a cut, apply a sterile bandage and apply a little pressure until the bleeding stops. Usually, with small amounts of bleeding, clotting will occur within three minutes, ending the bleeding.

For a raw wound, don't use dry gauze because it will stick, and when you pull it off later it will take with it the clotted blood and allow bleeding to start again. Instead, use sterile petrolatum (Vaseline) gauze, or apply a sterile ointment and then cover with gauze. Also available are nonadherent bandages.

If the cut is deep and gapes open, you may do as well as your doctor does when he sutures or stitches if you follow this procedure:

After the wound has been cleaned and the skin is dry, apply one adhesive end of a small sterile Band-Aid, or equivalent, on one side near the cut. With your other hand, apply just enough pressure to hold the edges of the wound together so they just touch, taking care not to pinch them together too tightly nor touch the wound itself with your fingers. Then lay down the other adhesive end on the opposite side of the cut.

If you do this in such a way that the edges of the skin come together nicely, you may well achieve the equivalent of a professional plastic surgery repair. *Note:* Only close the edges of a fresh clean wound; to do this with an old or dirty wound will enclose the contamination and result in infection.

If the cut is on the face or another visible area, to be certain you have done the right thing you should see a physician. If necessary, he can insert small sutures in a way to avoid scarring.

When you proceed thus, in a calm and certain way, you will endow your child with a sense of security not only about the immediate accident but also for the sight of blood, for any injury, and for illness in the future. If, for example, the child should be involved in an auto accident in the future, it will be possible for him or her to calmly assess the injuries, personal and of others, avoiding the problems caused by crying and fainting.

This, of course, does not mean that you should have your children make light of accidents. They should become aware of hazards and be taught to avoid them.

But realistically, accidents are not always avoidable, nor are illnesses, and the confidence engendered by this "Look at the bleeding" approach will serve your children, and quite likely yourself, well. If your reaction to an emergency—even losing your auto keys—is one of panic, think back on your own life. How did you and your parents react at the time of your first injury? Make up your mind to calmly evaluate the situation and react productively when next faced with an unusual, acute problem.

Poisonings

Each year in the United States, more than a million cases of poisoning (85 percent of them among children) occur, leading to sickness and suffering for many thousands and death for several hundred.

And please note well: *Often matters can be made worse by following outdated, inaccurate first aid labels* on many potentially poisonous household products—*and even by following outdated and erroneous information in some widely used first aid manuals.*

Although much information about poisonings and how best to treat them has been obtained recently, the first aid labeling on many products has not been changed for years.

Note These Matters of Concern:

• The labeling on many alkaline household drain cleaners, oven cleaners, and products that contain lye prescribes, in case of accidental swallowing, use of vinegar or citrus fruit juice to provide a neutralizing effect. But the reaction of these natural acids with the alkali may increase gastrointestinal burning.

• Often, the final instruction is to follow the vinegar or juice with butter or a cooking oil, which is supposed to be soothing. But it is also a coating and concealer— and wrong since it interferes with the physician's ability to determine the extent of damage and what further treatment is essential.

• In case of poisoning with an acid-containing or acid-releasing product, even some medical texts still recommend use of sodium bicarbonate. But that carries the risk of blowing out the stomach.

• For people who swallow alcohol-based products such as antifreeze, there is a decade-old instruction to induce vomiting with a tablespoon of salt in a glass of water. But the Consumer Product Safety Commission has reported that *this could cause fatal salt poisoning*—and that it is not safe to use salt solutions to induce vomiting for any accidental ingestion.

• Should vomiting be induced after swallowing a product such as glue, paint, fondue fuel, or furniture polish containing a petroleum distillate? Labels differ. They probably should caution against inducing vomiting, but it is more essential to take another step: call a poison control center. Under some circumstances, if a large amount has been swallowed or the product also contains a dangerous additive, vomiting may be needed. But if done at home, vomiting of a petroleum distillate may cause some of it to be sucked into the lungs. In a hospital emergency room, precautions can be taken and vomiting or washing out of the stomach can be done safely.

What You Should Properly Do About Poisonings

First, consider it absolutely essential to be prepared— just by having two things always on hand—so you can be certain you are helping, not hurting:

1. An ounce bottle of syrup of ipecac, which your druggist can sell without prescription.
2. The phone number of the nearest poison control center. There are now some 600 centers across the country. You may find the number of the nearest in the front section of your telephone directory. If not, ask your physician.

A safe first aid procedure is to give one or two glasses of water to dilute the poison. Then, immediately call the poison control center—or a physician, hospital, or rescue unit. Be prepared to report as much as you can about what was swallowed: name of product, maker, contents if they are listed on the container. And, very important, how much was swallowed.

You may then be instructed, depending upon the nature of the poison, to induce vomiting.

To make a patient vomit, give one tablespoonful ($1/2$ ounce) of syrup of ipecac for a child a year of age or older, plus at least one cup of water. If no vomiting occurs in 20 minutes, repeat once only. Keep the patient walking, and if no vomiting has occurred within 10 minutes after the second dose of ipecac, try to induce vomiting by tickling the back of the throat. In the case of a child, when vomiting does occur, place in a "spanking position" with head lower than hips to avoid inhalation of vomitus.

If syrup of ipecac is not available, try to induce vomiting by tickling the back of the throat with a spoon handle or other blunt object after giving water. But don't waste time waiting for vomiting if it is delayed. Take the victim promptly to a hospital emergency room or physician, bringing along the poison's container with intact label. If the poison is not known, the examining physician will make judgments based on other clues.

Please note well: You will not be wasting time getting through to a poison control center for instructions. The centers carefully collect information about the contents of various products from manufacturers and, with this knowledge, are in a position to advise you on exactly what has to be done—at home or otherwise—in a specific case of poisoning. *Always, specific treatment is better than general treatment.*

If an eye is affected: Immediately wash the eye gently, using plenty of water (or milk in an emergency) for at least 15 minutes, with the eyelid held open. Call a poison control center, doctor, hospital or rescue unit and get the victim to a medical facility promptly.

If the skin is affected: Wash off immediately with a large amount of water. Use soap if available. Remove any contaminated clothing. And call for help.

If a poison has been inhaled: Get any victim who has inhaled such things as fuel gas, auto exhaust, dense smoke from a fire, or fumes from poisonous chemicals into fresh air. Loosen clothing. If breathing has stopped, start artificial respiration (p. 40) immediately. Don't stop until breathing starts or help arrives. And while doing this, have someone else call for help.

The Best Way to Prevent Poisoning at Home

Keep these facts in mind:

- Most poisonings involve children up to 3 years of age.
- The unpleasant taste of a potential poison is *not* a deterrent to a child.
- The most dangerous time is the hour before the evening meal—a time that one poison control center physician calls the "arsenic hour"—the time when a child is hungry. At this particular time, it may be a good idea to place cookies on the table for a child

to grab.

Currently, medicines make up 50 percent of poison control center calls. At the top of the list: aspirin, tranquilizers, sedatives, sleeping pills, vitamins. Cleaning agents account for about 20 percent; insecticides, about 10 percent; petroleum distillates (gasoline, turpentine, lighter fluid, etc.) about 7 percent; the rest includes plants and cosmetics.

Keep all such items, all inedibles, in their original containers. (A common cause of poisoning is transfer of poisonous liquid to soft drink bottles.) And keep such items out of sight and out of a child's reach, with all medicines locked away.

Teach children never to take medicine unless given by an adult.

Shock

Medical shock—which has nothing to do with electrical shock—is a potentially grave emergency. It can cause death from injuries and illnesses that in themselves would not be fatal.

It is important for you to have some advance knowledge of what shock is, when it may occur, how to recognize it, and what to do for it.

WHAT IT IS: Shock is a depressed body state caused by upset of the mechanisms that keep blood circulating properly to all parts of the body. Because of the failure in circulation, the brain, heart, and other vital organs are deprived of adequate blood.

WHEN IT OCCURS: It may follow severe injury, severe burns, infection, pain, bleeding, stroke, heart attack, heat exhaustion, food or chemical poisoning, broken bones, exposure.

WHAT TO LOOK FOR: Paling of the face.

Cold, clammy skin with drops of sweat on forehead and palms of hands.

Restlessness, confusion, apprehension, trembling, nervousness or unconsciousness.

Pulse weak, small, rapid—referred to as "thready."

Nausea or vomiting.

Increased breathing rate, usually over 20 breaths a minute; breathing may also be irregular and with some deep sighing.

Sharp fall in blood pressure.

WHAT TO DO: Keep the victim lying down (if possible with head lower than the rest of the body) to encourage blood flow to the brain. A person with a *head injury* may be kept flat or propped up, but the *head* should *not* be lower than the rest of the body; otherwise swelling of the brain may occur.

Raise the legs 8 to 12 inches, supporting them on blankets or anything else handy, if there are no broken bones. This enables blood in the legs to reach the heart and major circulation. If there is increased breathing difficulty or pain when the legs are raised, lower them again.

If there is any bleeding, stop it if possible (see BLEEDING).

Cover the victim only enough to prevent loss of body heat if the weather is cold or damp. Don't overheat.

Check on the airway. If there is mucus or vomitus, remove it. A victim who is unconscious should be placed on his side to aid drainage of fluids out of the mouth and help avoid airway blockage by vomitus. If there is no risk of such blockage and the victim is having difficulty breathing, place him on his back, with head and shoulders raised on a blanket.

Fluids by mouth have value in shock but should be administered only under certain conditions: if medical help will not be available for an hour or more; if the victim is not vomiting or likely to vomit, and is not unconscious. Fluid given to an unconscious or semiconscious person may flow into the lungs, worsening the condition. Nor should fluid be administered if the victim appears to have a brain or abdominal injury.

The fluid should be water, neither hot nor cold—best of all, water containing one level teaspoonful of table salt and one-half level teaspoonful of baking soda to a quart. For an adult, give about half a glass every 15 minutes; for a child under 12, a quarter glass; for an infant, an eighth of a glass or one ounce. Stop fluid administration if the victim vomits or becomes nauseated.

A physician overcomes shock by giving intravenous fluids, administering blood if needed, and treating the primary condition that caused the shock.

Anaphylactic Shock

This is a grave emergency condition—a catastrophic, allergic, whole-body reaction that occurs in a previously sensitized person when he or she is again exposed to the same sensitizing material. The material may be an otherwise valuable drug such as penicillin, a serum, an anesthetic, or a sting from a honeybee, wasp, yellow jacket, or hornet.

THESE ARE THE INDICATIONS: Typically, within 1 to 15 minutes after exposure to a sensitizing material, a sense of uneasiness, agitation, flushing; giant hives all over the skin; swelling over the entire body; difficulty in breathing; coughing; sneezing; itching; nausea and vomiting (less common).

Then, within another minute or two, signs of shock may develop; paling of the face; cold, clammy skin; sweat on the forehead and palms; weak, rapid, small pulse.

Subsequently, the victim may convulse, become incontinent, unresponsive, and die. Someone in anaphylactic shock can be dead in minutes.

WHAT TO DO: Immediate treatment with epinephrine (Adrenalin) by injection under the skin is imperative.

Any person who has displayed sensitivity to a drug, serum, or anesthetic should always make that fact known to a treating physician and would do well to carry some indication of the fact—a card, bracelet, etc.

Anyone known to be sensitive to insect stings should always carry a sting kit when likely to be exposed. The kit, which must be prescribed by a physician, contains epinephrine, hypodermic needle, a strong antihistamine.

If a sting kit is available, 0.3 to 0.5 milliliters of 1:1,000 aqueous epinephrine should be injected under the skin (following directions in the kit), without loss of time—if possible, at the very first indication of anaphylactic reaction. A second injection may be needed for a severe reaction. And the victim should be taken to physician, emergency room, or other medical facility as quickly as possible.

If no kit is available, then during the trip to a medical facility, spread of the insect venom should be slowed by continuous ice or cold compresses applied to the site and by use of a tourniquet above the sting. The tourniquet should be at least two inches wide. If a commercial tourniquet is not available, use a triangular bandage, towel, or handkerchief folded several times. Wrap snugly—not so tight, however, that the pulse cannot be felt. Loosen briefly every four minutes. In case of a bee sting, remove and discard the stinger and venom sac.

Abdominal Pain

What do you do if you suddenly develop a bellyache, perhaps wake up with it in the middle of the night? By studying this section before you have a problem, you will be familiar with possible causes and how to check on them and narrow in on the probable cause and what to do.

First, take a short medical history; ask the questions your doctor would ask if you were to call him. Look back a little: Did you eat a heavy meal or sizable snack just before going to bed, or were you at a party where you did more than your usual amount of eating and drinking?

If it's a youngster who has the pain, did he, say, go to a movie and gobble three boxes of popcorn and a chocolate bar and drink a lot of soda pop?

More often than not, sudden abdominal pain is likely to be from something you ate. If the pain is not extreme or localized to any one region but extends throughout much of the abdomen, you can try an antacid preparation or a glass of milk. Did you have a normal bowel movement in the past 48 hours? If not, use a suppository to induce one. Retention of stool is a common cause of abdominal pain.

Is the pain diminishing? If so, you are probably on

your way to recovery; give it a little more time.

Whether it occurs at night or at other times, abdominal pain can have varied causes, some minor, some not to be taken lightly. And you can often determine what is likely to be the problem by considering where in the abdomen the pain is located, its nature, and any other symptoms that accompany it:

• When the pain is in the upper abdomen and accompanied by other symptoms that may include nausea, heartburn, flatulence, belching, feelings of fullness and stomach distention, all developing during or after a meal, the problem can be indigestion.

• When the pain occurs first in the area around the navel (belly button), accompanied or preceded by nausea or a feeling of "upset stomach," and then the pain *shifts* to the right lower quadrant or quarter of the abdomen, the problem can be appendicitis.

• If you have had an abdominal operation in the past, a possible cause of abdominal pain is formation of adhesions leading to intestinal obstruction. Such obstruction may sometimes occur from other causes. Symptoms depend upon whether the obstruction is in the small or large intestine and whether it is complete or partial:

—Severe, cramplike pain around the navel area that may come and go, vomiting that is recurrent and eventually becomes fecal, abdominal distention, and inability to pass gas or stool can indicate complete obstruction of the small intestine. With partial obstruction, symptoms are similar but less severe, and diarrhea may follow cramps.

—Pain lower in the abdomen, less severe, with abdominal distention, and with vomiting developing later may indicate obstruction of the colon or large bowel. If obstruction is complete, constipation is absolute and gas cannot be passed at all. With partial obstruction, bowel action may be irregular, with passage of frequent small stools.

• If your pain is in the right upper quadrant of the abdomen and it is preceded or accompanied by abdominal distention and by nausea with or without vomiting, the gallbladder may be involved.

• In a woman, pain in the right or left lower abdomen, sudden and severe, and often accompanied by nausea and vomiting, may be due to a twisted ovarian cyst.

• A severe pain that starts in the lower abdomen and gradually extends upward to the right upper quadrant and middle of the abdomen, increasing in severity without relief, with the abdomen becoming tight and rigid as a board, can indicate peritonitis, possibly due to a perforated ulcer.

• When abdominal pain (which may be either sharp and knifelike or deep and dull) is relieved by passage of gas or stool, and when such episodes are frequent and accompanied by any or many other symptoms such as diarrhea or diarrhea alternating with constipation, nausea, heartburn, headaches, the problem could be irritable colon.

• When severe pain is in the upper abdomen, sharpest in the area about the stomach, extending to the back and chest, and is relieved when you sit up, it could be acute pancreatitis.

• Sudden abdominal pain or cramps accompanied by any or many other symptoms such as nausea, vomiting, gas "gurgling" in the intestines, diarrhea, sometimes headache, fever, muscle aches, and prostration can indicate gastroenteritis, which can result from "intestinal grippe" or "stomach flu" virus, food poisoning, or gastrointestinal allergy. (See Allergies.)

What to Do: Consider calmly what the possibilities are in view of the symptoms.

If the problem lies with something you ate and the suggestions noted earlier help, fine.

If you can be certain that another nonserious possibility applies and it is of transient nature and will cure itself, fine.

Otherwise:

1. Eat nothing.
2. Limit your fluid intake to small sips of water or ice chips.
3. Assume any position you find most comfortable.
4. Do *not* take a laxative or enema.
5. Call your physician after noting as much as you can about the pain and its nature, other symptoms, your temperature, and what you think may be possible causes.

Chest Pain

This section, like that on abdominal pain, is an important one to be familiar with in advance of the occasion.

Almost the first thought that leaps into the mind of anyone experiencing chest pain is that the heart may be involved. It may be, of course; real heart disease is a vast enough problem. But according to some estimates as many as 20 million Americans, most of them men and many of them young, are bearing needless burdens of concern and limitation of activity because, although they may have experienced some of the symptoms, notably chest pain, they do not have anything wrong with their heart.

We will consider the chest pains of heart disease and their distinguishing features and also chest pains that have nothing to do with the heart and what distinguishes them.

Angina: the Pain of Coronary Heart Disease

The chest pain that may accompany disease of the coronary arteries which nourish the heart muscle (called coronary heart disease or CHD) is known as *angina pectoris*—"angina" standing for suffocating or choking pain and "pectoris" referring to the chest.

The situation that leads to anginal chest pain is somewhat analogous to what happens when the fuel line of a car becomes corroded inside, its inner wall thickening with rust deposits so there is less room for fuel to flow from the gas tank through the line to the engine. Enough fuel may get through at slow or moderate speed on a level road. But when there's a hill to climb or the driver accelerates, the motor sputters for lack of adequate fuel flow.

So may the heart sputter, causing anginal chest pain, under some circumstances when coronary heart disease is present, for in this disease the inner walls of the coronary arteries are encrusted to some degree with fatty deposits.

Angina is not like a heart attack, in which blood flow to an area of heart muscle is suddenly blocked off completely or severely restricted, damaging that nourishment-deprived area. Angina represents protest by, but not damage to, the heart muscle.

Angina usually appears, as may a heart attack, during exertion—running for a bus, climbing stairs, playing tennis, shoveling snow. The exertion requires increased work of the heart, which a well-nourished organ takes in stride. But the increased effort, which calls for increased nourishment, is difficult for the heart when the coronary arteries can't let through more blood.

Angina, as a rule, is felt as a constrictive sensation in the middle of the chest which often radiates, or shoots out, to the left arm and fingertips. But there are variations: occasionally, instead of in the chest, pain appears between the shoulder blades, in the left arm or shoulder, left hand or wrist, in the pit of the abdomen, in the jaws and teeth, or even in parts of the right arm.

Anginal chest pain has other characteristics. Usually, it is frightening as well as painful, triggering a sense of foreboding and compelling the victim to stop whatever he is doing.

Moreover, an attack is usually brief, over in a few minutes. It responds quickly to rest and, as well, to a nitroglycerin tablet. If chest pain persists for more than 15 minutes, it is not likely to be angina. You can be reassured that no heart attack is involved if the pain disappears quickly, but diagnosis by a physician is still warranted.

Heart Attack Chest Pain

The chest pain that is the hallmark of a heart attack can range from a slight feeling of pressure to a sensation that the chest is being crushed in a vise.

If an angina victim suffers a heart attack and at first assumes he is having just another angina attack, he should soon realize otherwise. This time, rest does no good, nor does nitroglycerine. Typically, the pain persists for hours and does not subside until a narcotic such as meperidine (Demerol) is administered.

Almost always with the chest pain there is grave anxiety, a feeling that death is near. Commonly, the face turns ashen gray and a cold sweat appears. Often, retching, belching of gas, and vomiting develop and sometimes may make a victim think he is having a stomach upset. Shortness of breath is common. Sometimes, there may be palpitation—a sensation that the heart is beating abnormally fast and hard.

Some helps in distinguishing the chest pain of a heart attack from angina and from chest pains unrelated to the heart: It is less likely to be a heart attack if chest pain is below the nipple and to the left; if the pain is localized completely to the left; if the pain is sharp rather than a dull pressure or squeezing sensation; if the pain comes and goes; if the pain lessens when you lie down. If the pain persists for only one to five minutes, it is probably angina, not a heart attack.

What to Do for Angina

If you begin to experience what appear to be anginal chest pain attacks, based on the characteristics previously described, by all means see a physician for thorough examination and treatment.

Angina need not make an invalid of you nor seriously limit your activities. There are medications your physician can prescribe—nitroglycerin and others—which can be used safely and effectively not only to relieve angina but also to prevent recurrences. Other measures can help, including perhaps graduated exercise and change in diet and some practical changes in life-style.

What to Do for a Heart Attack

If you know—or even just suspect—you are having a heart attack, act promptly. The first hours and even minutes can sometimes be critical.

Ask someone to take you to the nearest hospital or call the rescue squad. And once you reach the emergency room, immediately tell personnel there that you may be having a heart attack and insist on being taken to the coronary care unit.

From the moment you suspect a heart attack, try to stay calm and avoid moving. Lie quietly; make no effort to get up or help yourself if help is on the way.

If you are with someone who seems to be having a heart attack, the most important thing you can do, once you have summoned medical help or are taking him to a hospital emergency room, is to talk to the victim quietly, providing reassurance, emphasizing that help is coming or he is on the way to it, and that he will be all right.

The fact is that while a heart attack can be immediately fatal, most attacks are not—and when a victim receives prompt medical care, the chances of getting well are very good.

Note: I have seen instances where an ambulance has reached a victim and very fine paramedics have done an electrocardiogram which has appeared to be normal and have then suggested that he remain at home. If this should happen in your case, don't accept the suggestion.

Insist that you would rather be taken to the hospital and play it safe. Be happy the electrocardiogram is normal— but, should it change, you are better off in a hospital where you can be closely monitored and treated immediately.

Other Chest Pains Unrelated to the Heart

Once you have eliminated the possibility that sudden chest pain is related to the heart, it can be helpful for you—in deciding what the pain is coming from and what you should do for it—if you know a few basic facts about the chest and its contents.

The chest, of course, is the area of the body extending from below the neck to the *diaphragm,* the large flat muscle that separates chest from abdomen.

The chest is enclosed by the *rib cage,* consisting of twelve ribs and the muscles that join them together. Outside the ribs are muscles that move the cage and other muscles that move arms and shoulders.

Within the chest are the *lungs,* one on each side; the *heart,* which lies in the middle and extends a little toward the left; in the back, to the left and lying on the spine, the *aorta,* the large vessel that emerges from the heart and distributes blood to the entire body through arteries that branch from it; and, lying slightly to the right side, the *esophagus,* a tube that is part of the digestive system, about an inch in diameter, extending from throat to stomach, whose sole purpose is to carry food and saliva from throat to stomach.

Lining the chest wall inside is a thin membrane, called the *pleura,* similar in appearance to Saran Wrap. The lungs and other organs within the chest are lined by a similar membrane. There are no pain fibers in the membrane encasing the lungs and other organs but there are in the pleura lining the chest cavity, and this lining does cause pain if it is injured, irritated, or inflamed.

PAIN FROM INJURY: This is common. Did you bump into something, lift your child or grandchild a bit overexuberantly, feel an unexpected twinge during a golf swing or tennis serve, or perhaps get hit in the chest with a ball or other object?

If your chest pain—no matter where in the chest it is located—is aching, dull, gnawing, and if moving the arms or bending or sitting or standing or lying in a particular position is painful, chances are your pain represents a bruised rib or a strain in the muscles between the ribs *(intercostal muscles)* or in other muscles attached to the chest wall that move the arm.

Take it easy for a time, giving the bruise or strain a chance to heal, and you may need nothing more.

SHARP CHEST PAIN WITH A DEEP BREATH: If, on taking a deep breath, you feel a sharp pain on either side of the chest, this can be due to a fractured rib if there is a known injury (SEE FRACTURES) or to pleurisy. With pleurisy, along with sharp sticking chest pain, worse on inhaling, there may be fever, cough, and chills.

SUDDEN SHARP CHEST PAIN EXTENDING TO A SHOULDER OR DOWN OVER THE ABDOMEN: Such pain, accompanied by breathing difficulty and sometimes, at the beginning, by a dry hacking cough can indicate *pneumothorax,* collapse of a lung. This occurs when air gets between the membrane lining the chest wall and the membrane surrounding the lung, preventing the lung from expanding with each breath.

Pneumothorax can result from a knife or bullet wound, a car accident, or other injury in which the chest is penetrated, allowing air to enter. It can also occur spontaneously, for no special reason, or sometimes as the result of an existing lung disorder such as emphysema or, rarely, tuberculosis. Spontaneous pneumothorax also can be caused by rupture of a small balloonlike structure *(a bulla)* on a lung, which is most likely to occur in people with emphysema but also can happen in otherwise healthy people (most often in their teens and twenties). It has also occurred during diving and high-altitude flying.

There is a dangerous form of pneumothorax—the only type calling for emergency treatment—known as *tension pneumothorax*. In this, a tear in the pleura lets air in but not out, acting like a check valve. As pressure builds, the lung collapses completely, making breathing very difficult. Tension pneumothorax requires quick medical help, which can be lifesaving. Air must be removed and this may be done with needle and syringe.

Air removal may be required in injury pneumothorax, along with treatment for the injury. A small spontaneous pneumothorax may require no special treatment; the air is reabsorbed in a few days. For a larger one, several weeks may be needed before all air is reabsorbed and the lung expands to normal; recovery may be speeded by treatment to remove the air. In any case, pneumothorax should have medical attention.

CHEST PAIN CAUSED BY THE ESOPHAGUS: Swallowing a hot liquid rapidly can cause chest pain because the heat is felt by nerves outside of the esophagus. Pain of an intermittent or chronic type can be caused by stomach acids "burning" the esophagus.

CHEST PAIN FROM A RUPTURED ESOPHAGUS: This is a rare but critical cause of chest pain. Awareness of it is important, since the chances of cure depend upon how soon the condition is recognized and treatment carried out. Each hour counts. You can make the diagnosis by knowing the following: The rupture, or perforation, of the esophagus may result from severe vomiting or efforts to vomit (retching), straining at stool, swallowing a foreign object such as a meat or fish bone, or a crushing injury to the chest. Along with constantly worsening chest pain, there is breathlessness, and sometimes shock may develop. The perforation must be closed immediately by surgery and antibiotics administered to prevent serious infection.

HEART-ATTACKLIKE PAIN FROM A DISSECTING AORTIC ANEURYSM: An aneurysm is a dilation or ballooning out of part of a blood vessel, most often the aorta, the big trunkline artery emerging from the heart. In a dissecting aneurysm, the inner coat of the artery ruptures, permitting blood to enter between the layers of the artery wall, splitting or dissecting the wall.

Chest pain is severe, often mimicking the pain of a heart attack. A dissecting aortic aneurysm is usually the result of atherosclerosis and occurs mostly in older people. But it may result at any age from a severe accident such as slamming of the chest against a car steering wheel or a hard fall on the chest.

Hospitalization as quickly as possible is required. Medical treatment includes use of drugs to lower blood pressure. Surgical repair of the aorta may be needed.

OTHER CHEST PAIN: Chest pain can occur as one of many symptoms in infections, such as lung abscess (along with purulent sputum, cough, sweat, chills, and fever) or pneumonia (with pinkish sputum that may become rusty, fever, shaking chill, headache, rapid and painful breathing).

As a chronic rather than sudden acute problem, chest pain may occur in cancer of the lung and other lung disease such as silicosis.

Note, too: Chest pain can be part of the simple, yet often alarming condition of aerophagia, or excessive air swallowing, which also can produce abdominal distention, palpitation, breathing difficulty, smothering sensations, and other symptoms.

Choking on Food or a Foreign Object: Applying the Heimlich Maneuver

Choking is the sixth leading cause of accidental death and the leading cause in infants under age one in the home. It is sometimes called "cafe coronary" because in the past such deaths in restaurants often were confused with heart attacks.

It was in June 1974, that *Emergency Medicine*, a publication for physicians, first published my description of a proposed method for saving the life of a person whose airway is obstructed by food or another foreign body.

The technique, to which others subsequently attached my name, is now known as the *Heimlich maneuver*; very quickly it received widespread recognition and use. In its fifteen years of use, several thousand lives have been reported saved. The technique is taught by many public and private organizations and agencies; more than 20 states have passed laws requiring that a description of the method be posted in eating establishments and in some instances also in schools. In some areas, state and county medical societies have induced food suppliers to print the details on milk cartons; and teaching programs have been instituted in many other countries.

The maneuver is *not* simply a first aid procedure. First aid is "what to do until the doctor arrives." Rather, the maneuver—or *Heimlich hug*, as it also is sometimes called—is a definitive treatment. It involves understanding how exactly to diagnose and know immediately when choking is occurring and how to treat immediately a condition that would otherwise be fatal within four minutes of onset. It is not possible for a mother at home or a choking diner in a restaurant to wait for a physician, paramedic, or ambulance.

For this reason, I hope you will read now, in advance of need, what follows. You can learn, quickly, the simple facts of both diagnosis and treatment.

Although the maneuver was originally conceived with the adult rescuer in mind, teaching of the technique in schools has resulted in children saving other children— and their parents.

In one instance, a mother was driving, with her children in the back seat, when she suddenly heard screams and turned around to see that one child was choking and had turned blue. She pulled over to the curb. By then, she found that her 8-year-old son was applying the maneuver to his 6-year-old brother; a piece of wax candy suddenly flew from the youngster's mouth and hit the windshield. The mother said she herself would not have known what to do.

In another instance, a 13-year-old, finding his choking mother lying unconscious on the floor surrounded by his younger siblings, saved her by applying the maneuver in the supine position.

There have also been many reports of individuals who have saved themselves by self-application of the maneuver.

Diagnosis of Choking

Before the Heimlich maneuver brought public attention to the frequency of choking deaths, many persons choked to death while observers thought they were having heart attacks. There is no excuse for that now that the symptoms of choking have been defined. It is virtually impossible, knowing these symptoms, to think that a heart attack victim is choking. A heart attack victim is breathing and may complain of pain.

Besides, 25 percent of victims of choking are children, who are hardly likely to be suffering from heart attack. And 90 percent of choking victims are seen to be eating when choking occurs.

The setting is a clue—not only in but also near an eating place. It has been shown that over 98 percent of persons falling unconscious and dying in or near a restaurant or dining area have choked.

THE 1, 2, 3 OF RECOGNITION:

1. A person who is choking not only cannot breathe but also cannot speak, because the airway is blocked so no air can pass through the vocal cords.
2. A choking person turns blue, because oxygen is not reaching body tissues.
3. He falls unconscious, because oxygen is not reaching the brain.

In the various teaching programs for the maneuver used by public and other agencies, people are taught what has come to be known as the *Heimlich sign*: grasping the throat with the hand to indicate choking—a signal to a rescuer for prompt application of the maneuver. Once there is universal knowledge of the choking sign, diagnosis should be 100 percent. When you see a person give the Heimlich sign, say "Are you choking?" If he nods his head yes, apply the maneuver.

But even without the sign, recognition of choking should not be a problem most of the time—in view of the inability of the victim to speak or breathe and the beginning of blueness even before the loss of consciousness that follows rapidly.

And even if an episode is not observed, anyone who is slumped over a chair or has fallen and is unconscious in or near any place where food is served is a candidate for the Heimlich maneuver. Delay, even to try CPR (see p. 42), may be fatal, as the unconscious choking victim is only seconds from death. Of course, if a person is unconscious, not in a dining area, and not breathing, the situation does not suggest choking and mouth-to-mouth resuscitation should be attempted immediately; any airway obstruction will be immediately obvious and the Heimlich maneuver should then be performed.

Basic Facts About the Maneuver

The maneuver avoids the problems with past approaches to handling choking. Inserting a finger or other object in the mouth in an effort to retrieve an obstructing piece of food or other item risks driving it farther down. Pounding on the back is inherently dangerous because it may wedge the material more deeply. The maneuver, as you will see, can drive the material only toward the mouth.

The basis for the maneuver is simple: Even in the midst of choking and inability to breathe, a great deal of air remains in the lungs—and if the lungs are properly compressed, the air can be driven out with enough force to pop the obstruction out of the throat and mouth.

That is exactly what the maneuver does. Actual laboratory trials with volunteers in which instrumentation was used to measure air flow, volume, and pressure have shown that when the maneuver is performed, it results in the expulsion of an average of about one quart (940 cc) of air from the mouth in a quarter of a second at an average pressure of 31 millimeters of mercury, sufficient to forcefully eject an object partially or totally obstructing the airway.

The maneuver can be performed when the victim is standing, sitting, or lying on his back. And you can perform it on yourself if that should ever be necessary.

How to Perform the Heimlich Maneuver

STANDING POSITION: Stand behind the victim.

1. Wrap your arms around his waist.
2. Make a fist and place the thumb side against the victim's abdomen—*slightly above* the navel or belly button and *below* the rib cage.
3. Grasp your fist with your other hand and press into the victim's abdomen with a *quick upward thrust*. Repeat several times if necessary.

Note carefully: You press your fist into the abdomen below the rib cage by bending your arm at the elbow. Do not squeeze or compress the chest; this can cause serious injuries. I like to emphasize this instruction by saying: "The victim's life in in your *hands*!" (Not in your arms.) A review from the Mayo Clinic noted that with CPR—which, unlike the Heimlich maneuver, requires pressure on the rib cage—ribs have been fractured and chests crushed, causing fatal internal injuries.

SITTING POSITION: When the victim is sitting, stand or kneel behind his chair and perform the maneuver exactly as for the standing position.

LYING ON THE BACK (SUPINE POSITION): When a victim has fallen, don't waste time trying to elevate him to standing or sitting position. Turn him on his back, with face upward, if he is not already in that position.

1. Face the victim's face, and kneel astride his hips.
2. With one of your hands on top of the other, place the *heel* of your bottom hand (the part of the hand near the wrist) on the victim's abdomen, slightly above the navel and below the rib cage.
3. Press the victim's abdomen with a *quick upward thrust*. Repeat several times if necessary.

SELF-ADMINISTERING THE MANEUVER: If you yourself are choking and no one is present to help, you can perform the maneuver on yourself. Many people, aged 10 years to 85, have saved their own lives in this manner.

Place the thumb side of your fist into your abdomen, below the ribs and slightly above the navel. Grasp your

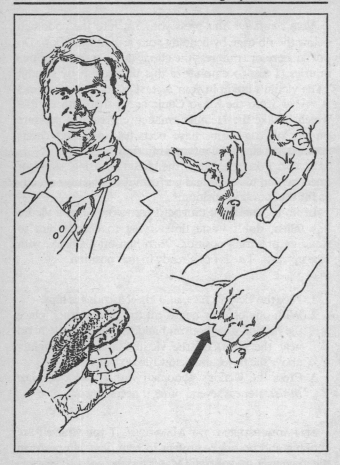

Fig. 1. Heimlich Maneuver. UPPER LEFT: The Heimlich sign. Hand to neck indicates: "I am choking!" LOWER LEFT: Making a fist (shaded area indicates "knob" to be used for pressing into abdomen). UPPER RIGHT: Placement of fist on abdomen. LOWER RIGHT: Position of other hand.

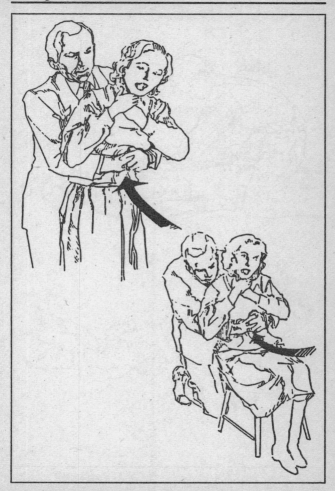

Fig. 2. Heimlich maneuver. TOP: For a standing victim. BOTTOM: For a seated victim.

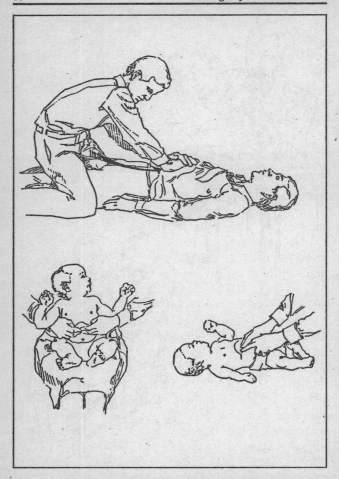

Fig. 3. Heimlich Maneuver. TOP: For a fallen victim or a small rescuer saving a husky victim. The rescuer uses his own body weight to perform the Maneuver. BOTTOM: For an infant.

fist with your other hand and press into the abdomen with a quick upward thrust exactly as you would do if you were attempting to save someone else. Or you can lean your abdomen against the back or edge of a chair, sink, table, even porch rail and press against it, applying pressure in the same place, slightly above the navel and beneath the rib cage.

SPECIAL NOTES: In 90 percent of reported cases, the maneuver has been applied from behind the victim, who was standing or sitting.

There are, however, two specific situations in which the supine, or lying-on-the-back, position is essential. First, as already noted, if the choking victim is unconscious and on the floor, no time should be wasted trying to stand or sit him up. Second, if the rescuer is too small or weak to reach around from behind, or if the victim is markedly obese, the maneuver can be performed only with the victim supine. Children have saved parents in the supine position, and petite wives their husky husbands.

It is essential in every case that the rescuer kneel astride a supine victim—never alongside—so that he can press into the middle of the abdomen and use the weight of his own body to apply enough pressure to elevate the diaphragm and compress the lungs quickly. Not only is the upward thrust less effective from the side of the victim, but it is impossible to apply the thrust directly in the midline. Inadvertent pressure to either side of the abdomen could rupture the liver or the spleen.

It is also essential, when using the maneuver on a supine victim, that his face be looking up; if the head is turned to one side (as may be necessary in other circumstances to prevent getting vomitus, blood, or water into the lungs, the throat will be contorted and a solid object obstructing the airway will not be able to pass through. If vomiting does follow the performance of the maneuver, you can then turn the victim's head to the side and wipe out the mouth.

FOR THE INFANT VICTIM: There are two ways to apply the maneuver to the infant.

You can hold him seated in your lap. Reach around and place the index and middle fingers of both hands against the baby's abdomen, above the navel and below the rib cage. Then press into the abdomen with a quick upward thrust.

Or you can place the infant face upward on a firm surface and perform the maneuver while facing him, again using index and middle fingers of both hands.

Common sense tells you to be gentle when performing the maneuver on an infant.

Artificial Respiration— When Breathing Has Stopped

Breathing failure has many possible causes, including drowning, electric shock, drug poisoning, chemical fumes, blocking of the airway by a foreign object, acute asthma, croup, and medical shock.

WHAT TO DO: Examine the victim's mouth and throat; remove any foreign matter.

Check for any indications of breathing: movement of chest, air coming from nose or mouth. Check the wrist for a pulse. If there is neither breathing nor pulse, go to CPR (cardiopulmonary resuscitation). If the victim is not breathing but you feel a pulse, indicating the heart is still beating, apply mouth-to-mouth artificial respiration.

1. Lay the victim on his back. Place one hand under his neck, lift up on the neck, use the heel of your other hand on his forehead to tilt the head back, thus opening the air passage.

2. Put your mouth, wide open, around the victim's open mouth, pinch his nostrils shut, and blow hard enough so his chest rises. If a small child is the victim, place your mouth over the child's mouth *and* nose while blowing.

3. When the victim's chest has expanded, stop blowing, remove your mouth, listen for the sound of exhaled air, and look for the chest to fall. Repeat the blowing and exhalation cycle.

4. If there is no air exchange, check the victim's mouth again. His tongue may be blocking the air passage. If there is still no air exchange, a foreign body deep in the air passage may be causing obstruction. With the victim still on his back, face upward, kneel astride his hips facing him, and use the Heimlich maneuver to expel the object. To do this, place one of your hands on top the other, set the heel of the bottom hand on the abdomen, slightly above the navel or bellybutton and below the rib cage. Press into the abdomen with a quick upward thrust. Repeat several times.

5. After the foreign body has been expelled, if the victim still is not breathing, begin mouth-to-mouth breathing again. Blow one vigorous breath every five seconds for an adult. For a child, blow smaller, less vigorous breaths every three seconds.

6. Don't stop. Keep up the artificial respiration until the victim begins to breathe. Many people have resumed breathing after several hours.

7. Have a physician or ambulance summoned as soon as you can. When breathing resumes, use blankets or coats under and over the victim to keep him warm.

Note: Many thousands of people have had surgical removal of part or all of their larynxes. They cannot use nose or mouth for breathing; instead, they breathe through an opening (stoma) in the windpipe in front of the neck.

When trying to help a victim of an accident or sudden illness, examine the front of the neck to see if there is an opening there (in some cases, a breathing tube may be worn in the stoma; if so, leave it in place unless it becomes clogged).

Use the same procedures as for mouth-to-mouth resuscitation but place your mouth over the stoma. There is often no need in this case to tilt the head back or to close off the nose and mouth. If, however, the chest does not rise when you blow through the stoma and the stoma is clear, the larynx removal may have been only partial and the victim may normally breathe through both stoma *and* mouth and nose. Tilt the victim's head back, close off mouth and nose, and blow again through the stoma.

CPR (Cardiopulmonary Resuscitation)— When Breathing and Heart Stop

CPR, meant for use when there is no breathing and the heart has stopped (as indicated by a lack of pulse), includes closed-chest heart massage as well as mouth-to-mouth respiration.

CPR can be lifesaving. But if used unnecessarily and incorrectly it can be devastating.

Closed-chest heart massage always carries some degree

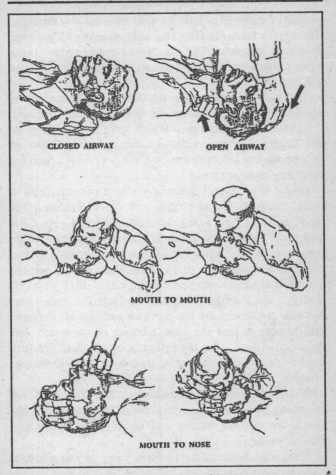

CLOSED AIRWAY

OPEN AIRWAY

MOUTH TO MOUTH

MOUTH TO NOSE

Fig. 4. Cardiopulmonary resuscitation. TOP: Establishing an open airway. MIDDLE: Mouth-to-mouth breathing. BOTTOM: Mouth-to-nose breathing.

of risk of causing serious internal injuries—by crushing the chest or fracturing ribs that may puncture lungs, liver, stomach, or spleen. The risk is very much worth taking when CPR is essential in a situation where life otherwise will be lost.

The risk is greatly reduced when the procedure is applied expertly by someone who has had training through a special course in which there is manikin practice. Such a course provides skill that cannot be imparted in a book. But information on CPR is provided here for desperate emergency use.

Please note: Don't mistake unconsciousness from a faint, choking, diabetic coma, or other condition for heart and breathing arrest. It could be tragic to use CPR and cause injury—especially if you are not expert in its use—in such conditions for which it is of no value. If you are in or adjacent to a dining area, there is a 98 percent chance that the unconscious victim has choked on food, and you must immediately do the Heimlich maneuver. *Do now read* carefully the previous sections on CHOKING and POISONING and the later sections on FAINTNESS AND FAINTING, STROKE, also the information on skull fracture in the section on FRACTURES, DISLOCATIONS, SPRAINS AND STRAINS.

WHAT TO DO: After first making certain there is neither breathing nor heartbeat (no pulse at the wrist), quickly check the victim's mouth and throat and remove any foreign matter.

Then you and someone to assist you—or you alone, if necessary—proceed thus:

1. Feel the victim's chest to locate the lower tip of the breastbone. Pressure must not be applied here or

the liver may be injured. Instead, find a point three fingerbreadths above the tip of the breastbone. Place one finger at that point and position the heel of the second hand next to the finger. Then place the heel of the first hand on top. Your fingers should be intertwined and lifted off the chest.

2. Push down with a quick thrust, using the weight of the upper part of your body to achieve sufficient force to press the lower portion of the breastbone down 1½ to 2 inches in an adult. Then lift your weight. Repeat the compression rhythmically once a second. If you have not been trained in the technique, remember, again, the danger of crushing the chest if you press too hard.

3. Mouth-to-mouth breathing also must be used. If you have no one to assist you, give 15 chest compressions and then stop in order to administer 2 deep mouth-to-mouth breaths. Keep up the 15 compressions to 2 mouth-to-mouth breaths until help arrives.

If an assistant is available, have him administer mouth-to-mouth respiration at the rate of 12 times a minute— once for every 5 compressions that you administer.

4. Continue the complete CPR (chest compression and mouth-to-mouth breathing) until the victim begins to breathe, pulse returns, and color improves. Do *not* give up after just a few minutes. Life can be maintained by CPR for an hour or more.

Note: If you would like to become expert in administering CPR, courses of instruction may be offered in your community. I cannot vouch for the success of CPR because the reports of its use are confusing. The method is reported here because it is so widely talked about, and its mention here does not necessarily indicate that I

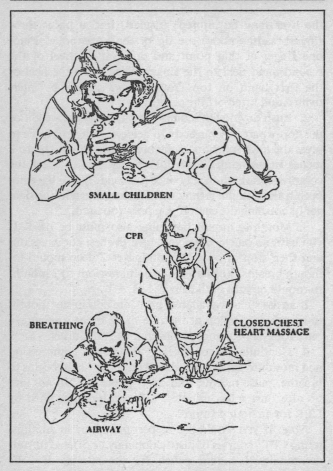

Fig. 5. Cardiopulmonary resuscitation. TOP: Mouth-to-mouth-and-nose breathing for a small child. BOTTOM: Mouth-to-mouth breathing and closed-chest heart massage.

endorse its use.

Burns

Burns can range from the relatively trivial, even if painful, to the devastating and life-threatening. And there are three factors to consider in determining how serious a burn is, what treatment to use, and whether medical attention is urgent. Those factors are

1. The class or degree of burn—essentially, a matter of depth
2. The extent—how much area is involved
3. The location

DEGREES: In a *first*-degree burn—which may result from sun exposure, light contact with a hot object, or brief scalding by hot water or steam—only the outer surface of the skin is involved. The skin is red, dry, painful, sensitive to touch, mildly swollen.

A *second*-degree burn produces redness or mottling, blisters, weeping and wetness, swelling, and pain. The burn has penetrated deeper into lower layers of the skin. The blistering results from bubbling of blood plasma through the damaged layers. A second-degree burn may result from severe sunburn, a flash from gasoline or kerosene, a spill of boiling water on the skin.

A *third*-degree burn involves not only the outer and deeper layers of the skin but also tissue below the skin. The skin is usually either pale white or charred black. It is swollen. Often underlying tissues are exposed. A third-degree burn may result when clothes are ignited or there is exposure to a flame, an electrical current, or hot object. Length of exposure and degree of heat are important in determining the amount of tissue destroyed. Often, because pain nerves are destroyed, there may be no severe local pain in the burn area, but the margin of the burn may be painful.

EXTENT OF BURN: Determining the extent is important because in an adult who suffers burns of 15 percent or more of the body surface—in a child, 10 percent or more—there is likely to be shock (see previous section on SHOCK). Any burned person showing symptoms of impending shock should be taken to a hospital.

You can roughly estimate the extent of a burn in this way: Figure that the surface area of a hand (both sides) equals about 1 percent of total skin area. Alternatively, you can figure in an average adult, the head has 9 percent of total skin surface; each arm, 9 percent; each leg, 18 percent; front and back of the trunk, 18 percent each; neck, 1 percent.

LOCATION: When the face is burned, there may be injury to the breathing passages, and as respiratory tissues swell, breathing may become obstructed. If the victim has difficulty speaking, swallowing or breathing, or is hoarse or wheezing, hospitalization is usually needed.

Burns involving the area around the eyes should be examined immediately by an eye doctor.

Second- or third-degree burns of the hand or any joint (elbow, knee, shoulder, etc.) should always be seen by a physician because contracting scars can develop later and interfere with function and movement.

WHAT TO DO: Remove clothing over the burned area immediately to prevent further burning.

For a first-degree burn, apply cold water or immerse

the burned area in cold water. If the burn is dirty, wash gently with soapy water, then flush with large amounts of cold water. Cooling can provide substantial relief and may speed recovery. If necessary, apply a dry dressing. If no complications occur, a first-degree burn should be comfortable within 12 to 24 hours and healed in about a week.

For a second-degree burn, immerse the burned area in cold water until pain subsides. Apply clean cloths wrung out in ice water for as long as an hour. Then gently blot the area dry. Do *not* break blisters and do *not* apply antiseptic sprays, ointments, etc. Apply a layer of non-adherent, light impregnated gauze such as sterile petrolatum gauze (obtainable in most drugstores) and hold in place with dry sterile gauze and a loosely wrapped bandage. If an arm or leg is burned, keep it elevated. Change the dressing next day and about every two days after that. If fever develops or if pain and swelling increase, an infection is likely to be present and antibiotic treatment may be necessary. A physician should be consulted.

For a third-degree burn, medical help is needed immediately. Infection may set in, healing is slow, scars can occur, and surgery may be required. Usually, too, intravenous fluids and treatment for shock are needed.

If the victim of a third-degree burn can be transported to a hospital immediately or medical help will arrive very quickly, make the victim as comfortable as possible. If the hands are burned, keep them above the level of the heart; elevate burned feet or legs. If the face is burned, prop up the victim and watch continuously for any breathing difficulty; if any develops, maintain an open airway (see p. 40).

If medical help will be delayed, remove clothing but do not remove any adhered particles of charred garments. Do *not* apply ointments, grease, other remedies or commercial preparations. Cover the burn with sterile dressings of clean household linen. You may simply have the patient lie on a clean sheet and loosely cover him with a second sheet.

Do *not* apply ice water to or immerse a large burned area; that may intensify shock. But a cold pack can be used on the face.

If the victim is conscious and not vomiting, have him slowly sip a weak solution of salt and soda, neither hot nor cold, made with one level teaspoonful of table salt and one-half level teaspoonful of baking soda to a quart of water. Give about half a glass over a 15-minute period to an adult, a quarter glass to a child, about an eighth glass to an infant. Stop fluid if vomiting occurs.

Chemical Burns

Of the skin: As quickly as possible, wash away the chemical with water, large quantities of it. Use a hose spray or shower if you can. Remove clothing from involved area and continue flushing with water for at least five minutes. If there is a container of the chemical with first aid directions for that particular chemical, follow them after the water flushing. Apply a clean dry bandage and get medical help.

Of the eye: Every part of the body is important, but few if any tragedies are greater than the unnecessary loss of an eye. Accidental splashing of a chemical into an eye is a danger in a chemical laboratory—but it can also occur in the home. I recall a woman who poured a drain cleaner (lye) into her kitchen sink. It generated heat and pressure, shooting upward into her eye.

As quickly as possible, pour warm but not hot tap water from a pitcher into the eye, with head tilted backward. To do this successfully, you may have to hold the eye open with the thumb and forefinger of one hand. It does no good to pour the water on a closed lid. Hold the pitcher close to the eye to obtain a gentle flow. If it is held too high, the pressure of the water could cause damage. Continue this flushing for five minutes, and without delay arrange for transportation to an eye doctor. In the meantime, after the flushing, cover the closed eye with clean, dry dressing and bandage. *Do not rub the eye.*

Coughing

Coughing has a purpose. It's an attempt by the body to get rid of materials—fluids, mucus, dust, other substances—from the lungs, windpipe, or throat where they don't belong. An effective cough can be a powerful force, releasing a burst of air at speeds of as much as 500 feet per second.

Because coughing is often protective, it is not always wise to try to suppress it with anticough medicine.

And, in fact, it can be helpful for you to know how to work with your cough—to make it, if necessary, more protective.

SUDDEN COUGH: Commonly, a cough that comes on suddenly does so because food or liquid has accidentally started the wrong way into the lungs instead of the stomach. The food irritates the lining of the airway, triggering a cough as a natural protective mechanism.

Normally, when you swallow, several things happen

automatically. The opening of the airway to the lungs, called the *glottis*, lies just behind and below the tongue. And right above the glottis is a flaplike structure called the *epiglottis*, which is attached to the root of the tongue.

With normal swallowing, the glottis instantly moves under the epiglottis so the flap of tissue can seal it off (much in the manner in which a flap valve closes), thus barring entrance of food or liquid into the airway, leaving open only the food passage. So securely in fact is the airway sealed off that if you were to try to stop halfway in the act of swallowing to take a breath, you would find yourself unable to breathe until you complete the swallowing act.

But accidents happen. Occasionally, you swallow the wrong way—which is to say that the epiglottis fails to function effectively, possibly because you were talking, laughing, or eating too fast. A bite of food or a swallow of liquid then moves into the glottis and you cough explosively to blow the material out.

It's important that the foreign material be expelled, because if it were to reach a lung, it could damage lung tissue or cause lung infection.

The best thing to do when a cough comes on under such circumstances is to encourage it—and, if necessary, make it more effective when, as sometimes happens, it becomes violent but not effective.

So you need to know the simple steps involved in producing an effective cough.

The first step is breathing deeply to get a large quantity of air into the lungs. Then, the opening of the glottis to the airway is closed as it moves under the epiglottis. Now, for a fraction of a second, you stop breathing and the diaphragm and muscles of your chest are splinted or held still. Try this—holding your breath purposely by compressing the muscles of your chest as if to blow air out but tightening your throat to keep the air from coming out. (This is what a child does when he has a temper tantrum and holds his breath.)

In the next step, the chest wall muscles are suddenly contracted further, reducing the inner volume of the chest and compressing the lungs. At this moment, the glottis opens and air suddenly rushes out.

That's the process involved in coughing.

If you find that your automatic coughing is not effectively eliminating a foreign object in your throat or windpipe, take a very deep breath and give a deep forceful cough, feeling it come up from the diaphragm. To be most effective, try to breathe in deeply enough to be able to cough out two or three times in succession without taking a second breath.

CHRONIC COUGH: A chronic cough that is not effective can be disturbing as well as useless.

Let's say that your chronic cough is associated with bronchitis or pneumonia. There may then be much mucus in the lungs and air passages. The mucous membrane lining in the passages secretes a sticky fluid, *mucus*, which serves to trap dust and other particles in inhaled air. Also in the passages are microscopic, hairlike projections called *cilia*. The cilia, through a continuous whip-like motion in the direction of the mouth, carry the sticky fluid upward so it can be swallowed or expectorated, thus helping to keep the air passages and lungs clean.

When mucus is excessive, the cilia may not be able to keep up, and the mucus must be eliminated by coughing.

Similarly, the cilia may not be able to cope adequately if you have post-nasal drip and secretions from the sinuses drain down the back of the throat and into the bronchial passages.

So if you have an accumulation of mucus and your coughing, though chronic and repeated, is not bringing the mucus up effectively, go through the cough procedure noted above and your coughing may become effective. Steam inhalation often can be helpful, too, by decreasing the viscosity or stickiness of the secretions so they become easier to bring up.

By all means, do not be finicky about coughing up and expectorating mucus into a paper tissue. That's where it belongs, not down in your lungs and breathing passages, and, in fact, it is not healthy to swallow excessive mucus.

COUGHING BLOOD: Sometimes, after a violent sudden fit of coughing or with chronic coughing associated with a cold, allergy or bronchitis, you may see a small fleck of bright red or browning blood in the sputum.

This is not unusual and need not be alarming. The strain of coughing and/or the irritation of the airways caused by infection or inflammation can produce the same type of abrasive effect on the linings of the breathing passages as would scraping some skin off the surface of an arm, in which case you would also see a small amount of blood.

If, however, there is more than one episode of coughing up a small amount of blood, it would be wise to see your physician for studies that may include a chest x-ray. He may also perform *bronchoscopy*, using a lighted instrument to examine the air passages. Bronchoscopy, formerly somewhat difficult because a rigid metal tube was used, now is done with a very small flexible fiberoptic instrument and hospitalization is not necessary.

If you cough up a fair amount of blood—say, the equivalent of a teaspoonful of pure blood or more—that can indicate a possibly serious underlying condition; it may, for example, be the first indication of lung disease. Even though it is a first episode and occurs only that once, you should consult your physician about it, not necessarily as an emergency condition calling for immediate attention, but by the next morning if it occurs at night.

If you cough up a great deal of blood or repeated modest amounts, emergency medical treatment is needed. Try to determine, if possible, where the blood is coming from—whether from the lungs, from vomiting, or has come up from the stomach to the throat and been coughed up. This information will help your physician to initiate the proper tests and treatment.

Note: Sometimes, coughing up of a sizable amount of blood can be due to a nosebleed that occurs during the night and is not noticed while you are sleeping. When you wake, you may cough up the blood from the nosebleed. Similarly, a nosebleed that occurs while you are awake may sometimes cause blood to run down the back of the throat and be coughed up. Such coughing up of blood is relatively rare. Stop the nosebleed (see BLEEDING FROM THE NOSE) and have the cause checked out by a physician.

Medical Emergency Kits

Remember the last time someone in the family cut a finger or picked up a splinter, or your visiting Aunt Lizzie tripped on a step—and you hunted fruitlessly in the medicine cabinet jumble for needed supplies and had to end up rushing off to the drugstore?

Yours will have been no isolated experience.

Supplies for medical emergencies don't have to take up great space—but they deserve their own space. Take the time to assemble those supplies, before you need them. Do this now!

I am presenting here suggestions for basic kits for the home and for the car and suggestions, too, for what to take with you for ordinary travel and also for a hunting, fishing, or other trip which may take you where medical help may not be close at hand.

Except where specifically noted otherwise, the suggested items can be obtained without prescription.

You should not put your home supplies in with other items in the medicine cabinet. Instead, keep them separately in a labeled container, which can be an old tackle box or small tool chest with hinged cover, or anything else suitable. Keep emergency supplies for the car in a similar container.

Keep the home container unlocked, on a shelf beyond a tot's reach.

Basic Home Kit

Sterile gauze dressings, individually wrapped, in 2- × 2-inch and 4- × 4-inch sizes, for cleaning and covering wounds

Piece of an old bedsheet, clean, folded, for use in making bandages and slings and in tying on splints

Roll of 2-inch gauze bandage, for securing dressings over wounds

Roll of half-inch-wide adhesive tape

Cotton applicators, small package, for removing foreign body from the eye

Feminine napkins, four, useful for staunching heavy bleeding anywhere on the body

Rubbing alcohol (isopropyl, 70%), small bottle, for sterilizing instruments and for sponging the body during high fever

Calamine lotion, small bottle, for insect bites, rashes, sunburn, etc.

Syrup of ipecac, 1 oz bottle, to induce vomiting in case of poisoning

Activated charcoal, useful for flatulence (gas)

Tube of petroleum jelly (petrolatum)

Band-Aids or equivalent, assorted sizes

Aromatic spirits of ammonia, small bottle

Aspirin or acetaminophen

Mild, nonstinging antiseptic such as Merthiolate, Zephiran Chloride, or Betadine

Milk of magnesia

Rectal and oral thermometers

Tweezers

Scissors with blunt tips, for cutting tape and gauze

Thick, blunt needle for removing splinters

Tongue depressors, for small splints

Basic Kit for the Car

Table salt and baking soda, 1 small package each

Matches, box

Bottle of distilled water, for burns and washing wounds

Sterile gauze dressings, individually wrapped, in 2- × 2-inch and 4- × 4-inch size

Piece of an old bedsheet, clean, folded

Roll of 2-inch gauze bandage
Roll of half-inch-wide adhesive tape
Cotton applicators, small package
Feminine napkins, four
Rubbing alcohol
Tube of petroleum jelly (petrolatum)
Band-Aids or equivalent, assorted sizes
Aromatic spirits of ammonia, small bottle
Aspirin or acetaminophen
Mild, nonstinging antiseptic such as Merthiolate, Zephiran Chloride, or Betadine
Tweezers
Scissors with blunt tips
Thick, blunt needle

Basic Kit for Travel

Steristrips, for use (instead of sutures) in holding together the cut edges of a laceration
Oral antibiotic for infections, prescribed by your physician
Marezine or Dramamine tablets, for motion sickness
Kaopectate, for diarrhea
Pepto-Bismol, for treatment and prevention of traveler's diarrhea (turista) if you go to a developing country
Doxycycline, an antibiotic your physician can prescribe, for preventing diarrhea (turista) if you go to a developing country
Sterile gauze dressings, individually wrapped, 2- × 2-inch and 4- × 4-inch sizes
Roll of 2-inch gauze bandage
Roll of half-inch-wide adhesive tape
Cotton applicators, small package

Tube of petroleum jelly (petrolatum)
Rectal and oral thermometers
Aromatic spirits of ammonia, small bottle
Tweezers
Band-Aids or equivalent, assorted sizes
Aspirin or acetaminophen
(If you use reading glasses, it would be advisable to take
    along, in case of loss, inexpensive eyeglasses with
    simple magnifying lenses, obtainable at "five-and-
    dime" and other stores)

Basic Kit for Travel to Isolated Areas

In addition to the items just listed for ordinary travel, it
would be advisable to add:

    Snakebite kit
    Suturing equipment

ABOUT SUTURING EQUIPMENT AND SUTURING: It would
be advisable to check with your physician for additional
advice and perhaps some basic instruction he may be
willing to give you.

A sterile suture package is available, with nylon
thread joined to the end of a needle. Size 3-0 suture
thread is generally useful except for the face; 5-0, which
is finer, is less likely to leave a scar.

The needle can be held with a *hemostat*—a clamplike
instrument that amounts to a small, self-locking, needle-
nosed plier, which also has some usefulness in removing
thorns and fishhooks, and even on occasion for repairing
fishing and other equipment.

Suturing may be necessary only when a wound gapes
so much that it cannot be treated any other way. In most
cases, but not all, the wound edges can be brought

together and held with a Steristrip. A deep cut in an area of the body subject to much movement sometimes can be a problem.

When suturing appears to be essential, clean the wound with soap and water, then dry it.

Holding the needle with the hemostat, take a stitch through the skin only, never beyond into fat or muscle. The skin is never more than a quarter of an inch thick. By staying within the skin, you penetrate no vital structure. If you should hit a blood vessel, pull the suture through and out, and start again in a site just a little above or below. Bleeding will stop if you apply pressure for a minute or so.

After taking the stitch, tie the thread with three knots. Cut off the extra thread, leaving the stitch ends about a quarter of an inch long to help remove them in about seven days.

Although there is some pain during suturing, it is not agonizing and lasts for only a second or two.

Avoid suturing near an eyelid since the skin may be distorted during healing, causing trouble later.

Part Two

An Alphabetical, Cross-Referenced Guide to Emergency Medical Situations

Abrasions (Scrapes)

These skin wounds, usually the result of scraping or rubbing, are shallow and do not go below the skin. But they can be painful, sometimes more so than cuts. Often, in addition to oozing of blood, many nerve endings are exposed, which is why the pain is severe.

WHAT TO DO: Take care to remove any splinters or foreign objects that may be embedded in the skin—and to guard against infection.

For removing objects, clean tweezers (dipped in alcohol for five minutes) are useful.

Thoroughly wash the wound with warm water and soap; this is most important. A bath or shower may be the best way to cleanse the wound.

You can cover with a sterile dressing if the wound is extensive, but this is not often necessary unless there is continued oozing of blood. It is best to use a non-adherent dressing—one that will not stick to the open area of skin.

If infection develops, it will not necessarily be obvious for 24 hours or so. Keep an eye out for any fever, pus, marked swelling, or redness. Swollen, tender glands (lymph nodes) in the armpit or groin also indicate infection. Redness about the edges of the abrasion is no cause for alarm but is part of the normal healing process.

If infection does develop, see a physician. Also see a physician if you are unable to get all the debris out from under the skin since, if left, it may lead to permanent discoloration. If the abrasion is extensive, and especially if there is debris under the skin, a tetanus injection may be wise.

Allergies

An allergy is an unusual reaction in one person to a substance that is generally harmless for most other people. Foods, drugs, substances in air, pet danders, clothing, jewelry, cosmetics, even temperature can be *allergens* (substances provoking allergic reactions) for those sensitive to them. Well over 20 million Americans have one form of allergy or another.

Usually medical help will be needed to determine the cause of an allergy and provide treatment for it. But there are situations in which you may be able to detect the culprit yourself and avoid it or take effective measures against it. If you have a known severe allergy, you may need to be prepared to treat it as an emergency by carrying appropriate medications with you.

Hay Fever

Capable of producing clogged sinuses, nasal stuffiness, sneezing, eye tearing, and general misery, hay fever can be caused by the pollen dust of trees, plants, and weeds.

Drugstores, of course, are well stocked with remedies. They include antihistamines such as Chlor-Trimeton Allergy Tablets and Syrup, Decapryn Syrup, Dimetane Elixir and Tablets. Antihistamines, in fact, are a mainstay of hay fever treatment, often offering rapid, temporary relief. Serious side effects from the drugs are rare, but a common complaint is drowsiness, which can be dangerous if you drive or work near machinery. Some people develop tolerance to the drowsiness after a time, and there can be some degree of difference in the drowsiness effect of various antihistamines for different individuals. It is also true that one antihistamine, satisfactory for a time, loses its symptom-relieving qualities, and you may have to search for another that may be satisfactory.

Oral decongestants such as Sudafed Tablets or Syrup are often used. They temporarily reduce swelling of the nasal mucous membrane, overcoming clogged nose. Although there are topical products—sprays and drops—they are generally best avoided for a problem like hay fever for which many weeks of treatment are needed. Oral decongestants are not as fast-acting but they have less addictive potential.

Some hay fever sufferers use antihistamine decongestant combinations such as Sudafed Plus Tablets or Syrup. Combinations are convenient. But with a fixed combination, you get dosages that may or may not be precisely right for you. And it is always best to use minimum effective dosages, as few times a day and for as short a period of time as possible.

If nonprescription preparations are not helpful, a physician may prescribe a more potent prescription product or use desensitization treatment aimed at building up tolerance through a series of injections.

Even if you do find a satisfactory nonprescription product, you should seek medical help at the first indication of a complication. Such complications include pain or popping sounds in the ear; pain above the teeth, in the cheeks, above the eyes, or on the side of the nose, indicating possible sinus infection; persistent coughing, wheezing, and difficult breathing, indicating possible asthma.

Perennial or Year-Round Allergic Rhinitis

This is similar to hay fever but may extend through much or all of the year rather than occur on a seasonal basis. Medical help is often needed for such allergy. But a recent study with more than 800 patients suggests that home humidification during the winter often can be surprisingly helpful.

Over a three-year period, the study found that with humidification such previous winter-long symptoms as dryness of the nose, throat, and chest were markedly reduced; breathing improved, permitting more restful sleep; the need to clear breathing passages of mucus in the morning decreased. Most of the patients, too, were free of respiratory infections during the winter for the first time in years. If you have a hot-air heating system, humidification can be achieved with a device that attaches to the system or furnace; if you have other types of heating, room humidifiers can be used.

Mold Allergy

Sensitivity to molds can sometimes produce nasal congestion, stuffiness, and other symptoms. Several measures are helpful for such sensitivity. Keeping dust accumulation to a minimum and eliminating plants from the home can reduce exposure to molds. A dry, well-ventilated and well-lighted basement also tends to discourage mold growth.

A measure that is often very useful—if it is possible for the family to be away from the home for two or three days—is to place a coffee can containing a small amount of formaldehyde in each room of the house. Left in place for 24 hours, the formaldehyde often eliminates molds for as long as six months. After its use, the house must be well aired. Formaldehyde is a dangerous substance; it should not be left in the reach of children.

Skin Allergies

Almost any substance coming into contact with the skin can cause redness, rash, and itching in those sensitive to it. But recent studies at ten major medical centers have identified leading troublemakers.

At the head of the list is nickel sulfate, often used in the making of inexpensive watches, earrings, rings, and bracelets. As many as 11 percent of those who wear such jewelry eventually experience allergic reactions.

Another major item is potassium dichromate, a substance commonly found in tanned leather, to which about 8 percent of the population is sensitive.

Common household antiseptics are also responsible for many allergic reactions. One, thimerosal (Merthiolate), can trigger attacks in 8 to 10 percent of users.

And an ingredient in many hair dyes, *p*-phenylenediamine, produces itching and other symptoms in 8 percent of users.

The solution to such skin problems is to suspect possible culprits, narrow in on the actual one, and remove it from contact with the skin. Often you can do this for yourself.

Drug Allergies

Although penicillin is the drug best known for causing allergic reactions—sometimes severe and life-threatening anaphylactic shock (see p. 16)—there are sensitivities in some people to other drugs, including tetracycline antibiotics, sulfa compounds, insulin, tranquilizers, and aspirin. If you are taking a drug that is new for you and develop an allergic response, you should call your physician without undue delay to find out if it is likely to be responsible for your allergic symptoms and whether it can be stopped safely and possibly a switch made to another drug.

A note about aspirin: As valuable as it is, aspirin is not well tolerated by about 0.9 percent of the general population. But if you have other allergy problems, your chances of being allergic to aspirin are increased— to 1.4 percent with hay fever or nasal congestion problems, to 3.8 percent with asthma.

Food Allergies

By far the chief offenders among food allergens are cow's milk, chocolate and cola (the kola nut family), corn, eggs, the pea family (chiefly peanut, which is not a nut), citrus fruits, tomato, wheat and other small grains, cinnamon, and artificial food colors.

Cow's milk—as important an allergen among adults as among children—may produce nasal and bronchial congestion, with excessive mucus production. It can also be responsible in some cases for constipation, diarrhea, abdominal pain, and distention.

Chocolate and cola may produce headache and in some cases are important factors in asthma, year-round rhinitis (running nose), and eczema.

Corn sensitivity may produce headache. It also can lead to allergic tension (insomnia, irritability, restlessness) and allergic fatigue (sleepiness, torpor, weakness, vague aching).

Egg may cause almost any allergic manifestation and is most likely to trigger hives and angioedema (giant hives, with sudden temporary appearance of large skin and mucous membrane wheals and intense itching). Egg also may contribute to eczema, asthma, headache, and gastrointestinal upsets.

In the pea family, the peanut is the most common offender. Mature beans and peas are more often problems than are green peas and snap beans. Pea family members can cause headache and may be involved in asthma, hives, and angioedema.

Oranges, lemons, limes, grapefruits, and tangerines may cause eczema and hives and are sometimes factors in canker sores and asthma.

Tomato is a relatively common cause of eczema, hives, and canker sores; it seldom induces headaches but may cause asthma.

Of the small grains—wheat, rice, barley, oats, wild rice, millet, and rye—wheat is the most allergenic, rye the least. Manifestations of grain allergy include asthma and gastrointestinal disturbances.

Cinnamon is a common cause of hives and headache and an occasional cause of asthma.

Artificial food colors are used in carbonated beverages, breakfast drinks, bubble gum, gelatin desserts, and many medications. The most important allergens among them are the red dye amaranth and the yellow dye tartrazine. Hives and asthma are the most common manifestations.

Other food allergens include pork, beef, onion, garlic, white potato, fish of all kinds, coffee, shrimp, banana, walnut, and pecan. Almost any other food can be allergic for some people.

Foods least likely to be troublesome are chicken, turkey, lamb, rabbit; beet, spinach, cabbage, cauliflower, broccoli, turnip, brussels sprouts, squash, lettuce, carrot, celery, sweet potato; plum, cherry, apricot, cranberry, blueberry, fig; tea, olives, tapioca, sugar.

If one food is suspected, it can be removed from the diet for three weeks; if symptoms subside, the food can be reintroduced to see if symptoms return. If several foods are suspected, all can be removed for three weeks. One is then returned, and later, at two-day intervals, the others are reintroduced to determine which one or several may be the troublemakers.

Cold Urticaria

In this little known but not rare allergy, the victim breaks out with hives, not because of a food, inhalant or chemical, but because of sensitivity to cold. Lips may swell and hives may appear when ice cream is eaten; hands may puff up and generalized hives appear when a cold object is gripped; hives may appear and there may even be loss of consciousness while swimming in cold water.

For this allergy, your physician can prescribe an antihistamine drug, cyproheptadine, which has been reported to produce good results.

Insect Allergies

The stings of bees, wasps, hornets, and yellow jackets can produce allergic reactions and sometimes dangerous anaphylactic shock.

Bites, Snake

Two principal types of poisonous snakes—coral snakes and pit vipers—are found in the United States.

Coral snakes occur from North Carolina through Florida, westward to Texas, and up the Mississippi Valley to Indiana.

The pit viper family includes rattlesnakes, copperheads, and cottonmouth moccasins and may be found in many areas of the country.

Pit vipers have a characteristic indented pit between eye and nostril on each side of the head. Their venom affects the blood circulation system.

The coral snake, a variety of cobra, is small, has red, yellow and black rings around the body, and black nose. Its toxic venom affects the nervous system.

WHAT TO DO: First, have the victim lie down quietly to slow blood circulation and spread of the venom.

If the bite is on an arm or leg, apply a tourniquet between the bite and the rest of body, using anything—belt, tie, rope, or strip of cloth—you can wrap and firmly tie around, but not too tightly. If properly tied, there should be some oozing from the wound and you should be able to slip your index finger under the band.

Stop a moment and consider: Is the bite poisonous?

A bite by a rattlesnake, copperhead, or moccasin will immediately produce stinging pain, rapid swelling, and skin discoloration. Later may come weakness, rapid pulse, nausea and vomiting, shortness of breath, vision dimness, and shock.

A coral snake bite may produce only slight burning pain and mild local swelling at the wound, but other symptoms will appear in a few minutes, including blurring of vision, drooping of eyelids, slurring of speech, drowsiness, sweating, increased salivation, breathing difficulty, and nausea.

If no physician is available and you believe the bite to be poisonous, sterilize a knife blade or razor blade with a flame. Make cuts through the skin at each fang mark—and also just a little lower than the fang marks where the venom is most likely to have been deposited. Make the cuts through the skin only and in the long axis of the limb. If you go deeper than the skin, you may sever muscles and nerves.

Then suck out the venom. If you have a snakebite kit with a suction cup, use the cup. Otherwise, use your mouth. Snake venom is not a stomach poison and you can spit it out and rinse it from your mouth. Suction is very valuable; if done quickly and properly, it can remove most of the venom. Keep up the suction for 30 to 60 minutes. If swelling begins to extend up to the tourniquet, leave that one in place but apply another a few inches above.

Thoroughly wash the wound with soap and water, blot dry, and apply sterile or clean dressing and bandage.

Get medical help as soon as you can for possible use of antivenin. If the snake has been killed, take it with you for identification.

Give no alcohol. If the victim is not nauseous and can swallow without difficulty, give sips of fluid.

If necessary, use artificial respiration (p. 40). Also, if necessary, treat for shock (p. 14).

Even if a bite has been by a nonpoisonous snake, check with a physician about possible need for antibiotic treatment and tetanus prevention.

Bleeding

Some bleeding—from capillaries, the tiniest of blood vessels—amounts to only an oozing of blood.

Bleeding from a vein—identifiable because the blood is dark red—is usually slow and even.

Bleeding from an artery—with the blood bright red in color—may be profuse. With each heartbeat, the blood may spurt from the wound. Arterial bleeding is much less common than capillary or vein bleeding because larger arteries are well protected within body tissues and not often subject to injury.

WHAT TO DO: You can almost always control bleeding, even when it is heavy, by proceeding calmly with certain definite steps.

APPLY PRESSURE: This works for minor bleeding and more often than not for even severe bleeding. And it is a preferable method because it prevents blood loss without interfering with normal circulation.

Apply a sterile gauze pad over the wound. If a pad is not immediately available, use a clean handkerchief, clean cloth, even an item of clothing, especially if the bleeding is heavy. When bleeding is profuse, rather than delay, use even your bare hand and worry about infection later.

Press the pad—or bare hand—directly over the wound. Most bleeding can be controlled by pressure. Once you have it under some control, apply cloth material if you have used your hand. A thick pad helps to encourage clotting of blood. A feminine sanitary pad is very effective. If you have already used gauze or cloth, apply additional layers. Then apply a tight roller bandage or cravat to maintain pressure. If you have nothing else available, use cloth strips or neckties.

Do *not* remove the bandage. If blood saturates it, add more layers of gauze or cloth and tighten the whole dressing over the wound. Take care, of course, not to wrap the pressure dressing so tightly that circulation is cut off.

Note: Clotting of blood is the body's means for controlling hermorrhage, but clotting may take as long as *three to ten minutes* so maintain direct pressure *for at least that long*.

ELEVATE: If no bones are broken, it helps to raise the bleeding part higher than the rest of the body. Because of the force of gravity, elevation tends to reduce blood flow to the injured site.

INDIRECT PRESSURE (PRESSURE POINTS): If direct pressure on the wound fails to stop the flow, indirect pressure—also called pressure point control—can be added. It consists of applying pressure to the artery supplying blood to the injury site. Remember: always compress the artery at a point between the heart and the bleeding site.

There are several points where that can be done, compressing the artery against a bone with your fingers or hand to check blood flow.

For an arm wound: Use the *brachial artery*. You'll find the pressure point on the inside of the arm, about halfway between the elbow and armpit, in the groove between the biceps and triceps (the front and back muscles of the upper arm). Place your thumb on the outside of the arm and press your fingers on the inside of the arm toward the thumb, using not the fingertips but the flat inside surfaces of the fingers.

For a leg wound: Use the *femoral artery*. The pressure point is on the inner thigh at the crease of the groin. With the heel of your hand there, press against the bone.

For a scalp wound: Use the *temporal artery*. The pressure point is at the side of the head just in front of the ear. You may have to press on both sides of the head to gain control, as the circulation extends across the head.

For a cheek wound: Use the *facial artery*. The pressure point is midway along the jaw, between ear and chin.

For head and neck bleeding: Use the *carotid artery*. The pressure point is on the side of the neck below the jaw, just before but not over the windpipe.

For chest, shoulder, or armpit bleeding: Use the *subclavian artery*. Press with your thumb in the groove behind the collarbone.

Note: Even the most severe hemorrhage will likely be controlled by a combination of pressure dressing at the wound site and indirect pressure at the pressure point for the supplying artery—*if the pressure is maintained long enough to permit clotting*.

ONLY AS A LAST RESORT: A TOURNIQUET: Tourniquets are rarely needed. They are used much too often, and they can be dangerous.

If you use a tourniquet, it should be only as a last resort to save life, with an understanding that what is involved may be the sacrifice of a limb to save life. When a tourniquet is applied, circulation to all points below it is cut off. If the tourniquet is left on for an extended period, gangrene (tissue death) may follow and amputation may be required.

If a tourniquet must be used, proceed thus:

1. Use a tourniquet at least two inches wide. If a commercial tourniquet is not available, use a triangular bandage, towel, or handkerchief folded several times.

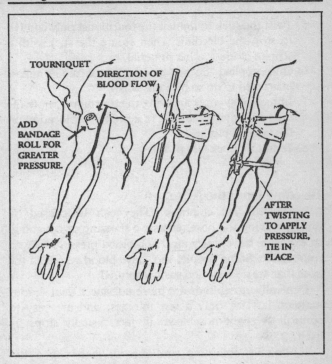

Fig. 6. Applying a tourniquet.

2. Place the tourniquet above and close to the edge of the wound. To be effective, as already noted, it must be between the wound and the heart.
3. Wrap the tourniquet tightly around the limb and secure it with a single knot.
4. Place a short, strong stick or similar object on the knot and tie two more knots on top.

5. Twist the stick to tighten the tourniquet only enough to stop the bleeding. Then secure the stick with a strip of cloth or other material.
6. Once applied, do not loosen the tourniquet unless instructed to do so by a physician.
7. Immediately after applying the tourniquet, note the time and attach the note in a prominent location on the victim's clothes.
8. Treat for shock (see p. 14).

Bleeding from the Nose

Nosebleeds are common. They can be caused by injury, picking the nose, excessive sneezing or coughing, or exposure to very dry air. High blood pressure may be responsible. Some people, too, have blood vessels in the nose that are delicate and easily ruptured.

Generally, nosebleeds are more nuisances than serious matters, last for only a few minutes, and are easy to control. A slight nosebleed, in fact, usually stops by itself.

If, however, bleeding continues or is severe, a few simple measures usually can be counted on to help.

WHAT TO DO: Sit upright in a chair and stay as quiet as possible. Do not tilt your head backward: keep it in normal position. By sitting up quietly, rather than lying down, you allow the blood to run out of the front of the nose rather than down the back of the throat. The latter could conceal the fact that bleeding is continuing; it also opens up some possibility that the blood may get into the lungs. Moreover, sitting up tends to lower pressure of blood in the veins, and if the bleeding from the nose is from a vein, which is most common, the vein has a better chance to collapse.

Apply pressure at the bleeding site by pressing the outside of the nostril toward the midline of the nose against the bony cartilage there. This is the equivalent of applying pressure to a bleeding site elsewhere in the body. And here, as elsewhere, if you maintain the pressure for at least three minutes—preferably a little longer to be safe—the blood can clot and bleeding stop.

Applying cold compresses or ice packs to the nose and face—especially above the nose or across the bridge of the nose—may help control the bleeding.

In the rare event that the bleeding persists more than 10 or 15 minutes or is obviously bright red and profuse (thus indicating that it is coming from an artery), maintain pressure on the nostril and do not let go until you can reach a physician or get to a hospital emergency room.

Note: If you have persistently recurring nosebleeds, they warrant medical attention to determine the underlying cause. Previously undiscovered high blood pressure may be involved or possibly some fault in the blood's clotting mechanism. These problems, or any others that may account for repeated nosebleeds, should and can be treated.

Blister

Generally, if a blister can be protected against breaking, leave it alone. The colorless, watery fluid will be gradually absorbed by deeper layers of skin and the skin will soon return to normal.

If the blister is large or in an area where it is likely to be broken—such as on the foot where it may be opened by shoe rubbing—follow these steps:

1. Gently clean the blister and the area around it with soap and water.
2. Sterilize a needle over a flame and use it to puncture the edge of the blister.
3. Gently press the edges of the blister opposite the point of puncture to force out the fluid slowly.
4. Apply a sterile gauze pad and adhesive.

If a blister has already broken, wash off the area carefully with soap and water, and apply sterile gauze pad and adhesive.

Bronchitis

Occurring most often in winter, acute infectious bronchitis, an inflammation of the bronchial tubes, may develop after a common cold or other viral infection of the nose or throat.

There may be the typical symptoms of a cold or other acute respiratory infection: chilliness, slight fever, malaise, sore throat, back and muscle pain, and profuse nasal discharge.

Onset of a cough usually indicates onset of bronchitis. At first the cough is usually dry and nonproductive, but after a few hours or days small amounts of sputum are brought up, and later the sputum becomes more abundant.

In a severe, uncomplicated case of acute bronchitis, fever of up to 102°F may be present for three to five days, after which acute symptoms subside, although cough may continue for two or three weeks. Persistent fever may indicate complicating pneumonia.

WHAT TO DO: Rest is important until fever subsides. Plenty of fluids should be taken. Steam inhalations are helpful. Aspirin or acetaminophen every four to eight hours relieves malaise and reduces fever. **WARNING:** Do not give aspirin to children as it is said to cause Reye's Syndrome, a life-threatening condition.

Expectorant drugs may be used. When effective, they loosen secretions in the air passages and increase expectoration. Actually, the proverbial remedy, chicken soup, as long as it has plenty of pepper, garlic and possibly curry powder, can be helpful for the same purpose. Do not let embarrassment cause you to permit secretions to accummulate in the lungs. The cough is nature's way of getting rid of the mucus. Cough it up and spit it out into paper tissue.

For a lingering, nonproductive, irritative cough, either a codeine or other cough mixture, or a vaporizer, can be used.

If you run a high fever and are more than mildly ill, if the sputum becomes pus-laden indicating a possible bacterial infection on top of the original infection, or if there are other complicating factors, you should consult a physician. A suitable antibiotic may be needed.

Note: Although bronchitis is commonly a mild disease in a normally healthy person, it can be serious enough to warrant immediate attention in someone who is elderly, is debilitated for any reason, or has chronic lung or heart disease.

Bruises (Contusions)

In a bruise, or contusion, usually the result of a blow with a blunt object, there is no break in the skin but small blood vessels under the skin are ruptured and the internal bleeding is manifested in the typical black-and-blue mark.

WHAT TO DO: Minor bruises heal without special treatment. Applications of cold packs or ice in a towel, though, will help diminish the swelling, reduce pain caused by the swelling, and speed healing.

In healing, as blood is reabsorbed, the skin color gradually changes over a period of about two or three weeks from blue to green to yellow to normal.

If pain persists for more than a day, hot applications—hot water bottle, heating pad, or a warm-water-soaked towel—can help (but do not apply heat in the first 24 hours, as it may increase swelling).

If a bruise is very severe or if the blow was very forceful and the bruise is immediately over a bone, there is possibility that the bone may have been fractured, and an x-ray probably will be needed.

Cuts (Lacerations)

Most of the time, cuts affect just the skin and under-skin fatty tissue and heal well without need for medical help.

WHAT TO DO: For such minor cuts, apply soap and water vigorously, and make certain no debris is left. You can then usually apply Band-Aids or strips of sterile paper tape so that the wound edges come together neatly and are held that way. Do not pull the edges together if the cut occurred more than three or four hours before.

When may medical help be needed?

If there are any indications of infection—pus, fever, marked redness and swelling (which, if they are going to physician should be consulted.

If there are any indications of nerve or major blood vessel damage—numbness, tingling, weakness (in a cut arm or leg), or vigorous blood flow—medical help is needed.

A physician should be seen if, for any reason, the edges of a fresh cut—perhaps because they are jagged—cannot be brought together neatly.

Unless very minor, any facial laceration should be repaired by a physician, perhaps even by a surgeon, so as to minimize possibility of a disfiguring scar.

Any deep laceration of the hand should be looked at by a physician because of the possibility that nerves for sense of touch or tendons controlling finger movements may have been cut and need very precise repair.

A SPECIAL WORD ABOUT SUTURING: There seems to be a common impression that suturing, or stitching, is the optimal way to repair a cut. That is not necessarily so. The only reason for suturing is to bring cut edges into contact so as to minimize scarring and promote healing or to control bleeding.

If a cut is not deep, if edges are not jagged and are close to each other, if no tendons, nerves or major blood vessels under the skin are involved, you can easily and effectively carry out the repair yourself by bringing the edges into contact and holding them there with tape or a few Band-Aids placed carefully across instead of length-wise along the cut.

But, by all means, in other situations, or if you have doubts about how effectively you are repairing even a minor cut, see a physician.

See also scalp laceration under HEAD INJURIES.

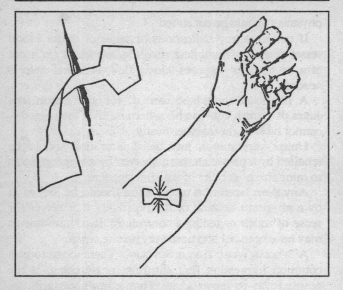

Fig. 7. Bringing edges of a cut together with tape.

Dizziness

Almost everyone has experienced the sensation of dizziness as a result of whirling around too fast or too long or perhaps while looking down from a great height. This sensation is markedly different from severe attacks of dizziness which physicians call *vertigo.*

It's important to distinguish the two if relief is to be obtained.

The first kind of dizziness is commonly described as a faint feeling, light-headedness, giddiness, or a kind of head-swimming sensation.

On the other hand, with true vertigo, you feel that you

are being whirled about or that everything around you is whirling. In addition, you may be pale and sweaty, feel nauseated and may vomit, and may try to stay in one place because movement makes the symptoms worse. Vertigo also may sometimes be accompanied by ringing in the ears *(tinnitus)* or uncontrollable movements of the eyes *(nystagmus).*

It is not unusual for dizziness to occur with high fever or under other circumstances: when you have not eaten for a long time, or have smoked excessively, had too much to drink, or even when you get up very suddenly from a sitting or lying position so there is a momentary lapse in adequate blood supply to the brain.

Vertigo results from a disturbance somewhere in the balance or equilibratory apparatus, which consists of the labyrinth of the inner ear, areas of the brain, and the eyes.

These structures may be affected by any of a variety of disorders. Infections in or around the inner ear may lead to severe vertigo, as may bleeding into the labyrinth. Medicines such as quinine, salicylates (aspirin and aspirinlike compounds), and the antibiotic streptomycin, as well as opiates and alcohol, may sometimes set off vertigo by a toxic effect on the labyrinth. Motion sickness is a frequent cause. Brain or ear tumors, middle ear infection, and skull fracture can produce vertigo.

Meniere's disease, which involves faulty functioning of the labyrinth of the ear, is marked by attacks of true vertigo. In addition, there may be ringing in the ears and hearing impairment. Attacks last from a few minutes to several hours.

WHAT TO DO: For an occasional attack of dizziness that is not true vertigo, you can try drinking a glass of orange juice. Also, make it a practice to take it easy when getting up from a seated or lying-down position. One of the nonprescription antihistamine drugs sold for motion sickness may be helpful.

If dizziness is a recurring problem, it would be wise to have a physician check your blood pressure and examine your ear canals. He may also suggest other studies.

For true vertigo, you may get some relief from an attack with bed rest and an antihistamine. But don't leave it at that. Medical help is needed to determine and eliminate the cause—and even as the cause is sought and treated, the physician may prescribe more potent antihistamine or other medication to provide more effective relief for symptoms.

Earache

If you have an earache, pulling on the earlobe may help indicate whether there is infection in the outer ear canal or in the middle ear. If pain is intensified by pulling, the likelihood is that the problem lies in the outer ear canal.

Outer ear canal infection can occur at any time of year but is most common in summer during the swimming season and is often called *swimmer's ear*. Some people, particularly the allergic, are especially prone to such infections. Injury from trying to clean the ear canal with cotton-tipped sticks and the like can predispose to infection. Actually, the ear has its own cleansing mechanism, and your cleaning attempts may interfere with the mechanism, promoting accumulation of wax and debris behind which water can be trapped, setting the stage for infection.

An outer ear canal infection can be localized as a

furuncle or boil or can involve the entire canal. If the entire canal is involved, there is likely to be itching, foul-smelling discharge, and sometimes some loss of hearing as well as pain. A boil causes severe pain and, when it drains, a brief pus discharge.

Infection of the middle ear, called *acute otitis media,* can occur at any age but is particularly common in children under 3 years of age. The first complaint usually is severe and persistent earache. In a young child, there may be little or no pain but the child may pull at the ear. Hearing loss may occur. And in a young child, fever up to 105°F, nausea, vomiting, and diarrhea may be present.

WHAT TO DO:

For outer ear infection, apply heat to the ear. Dry heat helps relieve pain and, particularly in the case of a boil in the outer ear canal, speeds resolution.

Get medical help.

For a boil, along with other treatment, codeine may be needed for the pain.

When the entire outer ear canal is infected, an antibiotic solution and, often, a solution of a corticosteroid such as hydrocortisone can be used, with the corticosteroid helping to reduce swelling in the ear so the antibiotic can penetrate all through the canal.

For middle ear infection, antibiotic treatment is often needed to relieve symptoms, bring infection under control and reduce the possibility of complications such as mastoid infection and damage to the hearing mechanisms. Among other often-valuable measures the physician may use are nose drops containing an agent such as phenylephrine to improve drainage through the eusta-

chian tube, which is a canal connecting the middle ear
and throat. Ephedrine sulfate or a similar drug may be
given by mouth, and if you are allergic, an antihistamine
may also be prescribed for a week or so to improve
eustachian tube function.

Faintness and Fainting

Fainting, in which consciousness is suddenly lost, usually results from an insufficient supply of blood to the
brain. It may occur as a reaction to fear, hunger, pain, or
any emotional or physical shock.

Prior to a faint, there usually are warning signs and
symptoms: extreme pallor, sweating, coldness of the skin,
lightheadedness or dizziness, nausea.

WHAT TO DO: To prevent a fainting attack, anyone
experiencing any of the warning indications should lie
down if a bed is available, with legs somewhat elevated
and collar and clothing loosened. Alternatively, sit down
and lower the head between the knees for about five
minutes. This will increase flow of blood and oxygen to
the brain.

Once a faint has occurred, the victim should be left
lying down, placed on his back, with legs elevated.
Loosen any constricting clothing. If the faint has
occurred indoors, open a window. Do not give any liquid
unless the victim has revived. Do not pour water over the
face because of the possibility that some may be sucked
into the lungs. Bathe the face gently with cool water. If
aromatic spirits of ammonia or smelling salts are available, hold them under the nose.

In several minutes, consciousness usually will be
regained. Keep the victim lying down for another ten

minutes, then have him get up slowly.

If recovery is not prompt, the problem could be more than a simple fainting spell and medical help is needed.

Note: Unfortunately, fainting has on occasion been mistaken for a heart attack and cardiopulmonary resuscitation (CPR) has been started when it was not needed. CPR is not entirely innocuous; it can produce injury; when needed, it can mean the difference between life and death; but its needless use may sometimes be tragic.

Remember

Remember these facts about fainting or "feeling faint" and you will be better able to handle the situation:

DIAGNOSIS:

1. The victim is usually well and without previous complaint (no pain, nausea, headache, etc.) but suddenly pales and loses consciousness.
2. The pulse is thready, feeble, or not detectable.
3. Breathing continues; signs of recovery occur quickly.

TREATMENT:

1. Have victim lie flat and elevate legs.
2. Loosen clothing.
3. Hold aromatic spirits of ammonia or smelling salts under nose.

DO NOT:

1. Give cardiopulmonary resuscitation (CPR).
2. Give any liquid by mouth.

3. Attempt to have victim sit up or rise.

Fever

One remarkable fact about fever is how almost anyone can sense its presence, even when the temperature elevation is only moderate. It is also a fact that fever accompanies a wide range of illnesses. And it is no less a fact that many people worry unduly about a temperature elevation that may even be normal for them. I know of one person who was deeply concerned when he forgot to take his thermometer along with him on a vacation.

Despite marked changes in air temperature, body temperature remains remarkably constant, within a range of about 1° or 1.5° Fahrenheit. Temperature control is achieved not only through the clothes you select but also by automatic dilation and constriction of blood vessels that carry blood to the skin and extremities—and by sweating which cools and shivering which increases muscle activity in order to generate more heat.

You should know that there is nothing sacrosanct about a so-called normal temperature of 98.6°F. Many people have normal temperatures in the range of 97° to 100°. Whatever the normal for an individual, almost certainly temperature will be lowest in the early morning, will rise during the day and usually reach a peak in the early evening.

Taking a temperature is simple enough. But you should know that there will be a difference between oral and rectal temperature. Rectal is usually half a degree to a whole degree higher because the thermometer tip gets closer to the central core of the body. Oral temperature is an adequate measure if the mouth is kept tightly closed while it is being taken—something difficult in children and adults who breathe through the mouth.

There is usually no need to worry about a temperature that does not exceed 100°F. Nor is there if the temperature is low unless it falls below 96°, in which case take the temperature again. If it still comes to less than 96°, better check to make certain that the thermometer is not broken.

Some more useful facts about fever: Your pulse rate will usually increase by about 10 beats a minute above your usual pulse rate with each degree of temperature elevation. If you should have fever associated with an infection, which is common, and your pulse rate does not go up, the likelihood is that you have a viral rather than bacterial infection.

Such uncomfortable symptoms as headache and chills, which may be associated with fever, usually vary in intensity. So does temperature level. Except mostly in some chronic diseases of long standing, fever rarely stays at a constant high level but goes up and down.

It's the variation in temperature that is associated with some uncomfortable symptoms, such as chills followed by flushing as temperature rises and profuse sweating as the temperature falls.

CAUSES: Almost any illness can cause fever. Any injury to the body may do so. Most often, fever is associated with infection, bacterial or viral. Usually, when fever comes on abruptly and there are also headache, respiratory symptoms or gastrointestinal upset or both, malaise, and muscle and joint pains, the cause is viral.

WHAT TO DO: Even now, there is some uncertainty and controversy among physicians about the advisability of treating or letting alone a mild fever—say, up to about 102°. There is some evidence that temperature elevation may be part of the body's defense mechanism against infections.

If temperature climbs higher, however, it should be lowered or it can be debilitating. In a child under 3 years of age, it is usually advisable to avoid letting fever go beyond 103°, for there is some possibility of convulsions (a reassuring observation from recent studies is that such convulsions rarely have lasting effects). And certainly, in older children and adults, if confusion or delirium is associated with high fever, the fever should be treated promptly.

Usually, aspirin* is the drug of choice, although acetaminophen can be used instead. In addition, when temperature is very high, sponging with cool water or rubbing alcohol will help. Sponge the entire body, paying particular attention to the armpits and between the legs.

Note that when aspirin or acetaminophen is used, there will be temporary relief of associated symptoms, but there may also be some discomfort as the drug brings the temperature down and then the temperature climbs again. For more comfort, aspirin* or acetaminophen can be taken about every four hours. Be careful, though, since the fever provides some indication of the severity of the underlying problem, and keeping temperature down constantly with drugs may mask increasing severity of an illness.

Fluid loss with fever can be substantial even if there is

---

*NOTE: *Aspirin must not be given to children since it can result in Reye's Syndrome, a life-threatening condition.*

no apparent sweating. So fluids should be given. Water can be used. Water, however, will not replace the vital chemicals lost in perspiration—and for their replacement, the old-fashioned idea of chicken soup has merit.

Obviously, the best treatment for fever is treatment of the cause if that is possible. With a viral illness such as flu, there is no curative drug, and home treatment (see INFLUENZA) is justified unless complications develop.

It can be especially important, if a child is the patient, to get in touch with the physician if the child has a stiff neck, rash, breathing difficulty, looks very ill, or is lethargic.

Fever Blisters (Cold Sores)

These itching or stinging sores on the skin or mucous membranes, known both as fever blisters and as cold sores, usually occur with a cold or fever, and are caused by a virus, herpes simplex. They may also follow exposure to sun and wind, a gastrointestinal upset, or even emotional distress.

They usually dry up after several days, form a crust, and clear within a week or so. Drying lotions or liquids such as calamine, camphor spirit, or 70 percent alcohol may be helpful, and can be applied with bits of cotton. During the onset period, cold cream may provide some relief. When the crust has formed, zinc oxide applied to it may speed recovery.

Fractures, Dislocations, Sprains, and Strains

There is sometimes confusion about definitions. To clarify:

A *fracture* is a break or crack in a bone. A closed or simple fracture is one in which bone does not cut through the skin. An open or compound fracture is one in which broken ends of bone protrude through the skin.

A *dislocation* is a separation or displacement of the end of a bone from a joint such as at the shoulder, elbow, finger, or thumb.

A *sprain* is an injury to the soft tissue about a joint. Muscles, ligaments, and tendons, which are attached to bones, serve both to move them and to hold them in place. In a sprain, the muscles, ligaments, and tendons— and blood vessels as well—are stretched or torn. The most common sprains are of the ankles, fingers, wrists, and knees.

A *strain* is a muscle injury in which muscle fibers are stretched and sometimes partially torn. A common strain is of the back due to improper lifting using the back instead of the legs.

Fractures

Bone fractures most commonly result from falls, automobile accidents, and injuries during sports and recreational activities. Sometimes, in an older person, because of bone brittleness, a break may result from only relatively slight injury.

RECOGNIZING FRACTURES: Some are obvious. The victim may hear or feel a bone snap or may be aware of broken bones rubbing together and producing a grating sensation. There may be a difference in shape or length of a bone on one side of the body in comparison with its counterpart on the other side. Or there may be an obvious deformity. Other indications of fracture include swelling, discoloration, and pain or tenderness to touch.

Often, however, not enough clear-cut indications are

the arm and secure with ties. Do not allow the splint to press into the armpit or it will interfere with blood circulation.

If the arm is bent, put it in a sling and bind it firmly to the side of the body.

FOREARM OR WRIST FRACTURE: Apply well-padded splints on each side from hand to elbow. Support the arm in a sling adjusted so the fingers are about four inches higher than the elbow (or a little less in a child). Leave fingertips uncovered so you can watch for any swelling or blueness; if either or both appear, carefully loosen the splint or sling slightly. If a doctor cannot be reached, at night remove the sling and allow the arm to rest on a pillow with hand higher than elbow.

FINGER FRACTURE: Immobilize the injured finger with a splint. Use a sling to support the hand. Keep the hand higher than the elbow, day and night.

UPPER LEG FRACTURE: With fracture of the femur, or upper leg bone, there is usually severe pain and disability. The foot usually is turned outward, and the limb is shortened because muscular spasm causes overlapping of bone ends. Watch for and treat shock if it appears (see p. 14). If the victim will be moved only a short distance on a stretcher, put a blanket between the legs, then bind the legs together. In this way, the uninjured leg acts as a splint. If it is necessary to use splints, pad them well. One splint should reach, on the outer side, from just below the armpit to below the heel; the other, on the inner side, should extend from just below the groin to below the heel.

KNEECAP FRACTURE: The kneecap, or *patella,* a small bone just in front of the knee joint, plays an important role in knee joint motion. When the patella is fractured, the pull of large leg muscles tends to separate broken fragments. Look for pain and tenderness at the fracture site, and inability to straighten out the leg. Sometimes, by gently running fingers over the kneecap, you will find a groove due to separation of the bony fragments. Gently straighten out the leg. The best splint is a board, four to six inches wide, long enough to reach from buttock to just below the heel. Pad well with clean rags or other material. Tie limb to board, leaving the kneecap itself exposed, since there may be rapid swelling. Check every 20 minutes or so to see that bindings do not cut off circulation. Loosen slightly if necessary. If no board is available, place a pillow or rolled-up blanket under the knee and tie in place. Transport the victim lying down.

LOWER LEG FRACTURE: Lower leg bones are the shin-bone, or tibia, which carries body weight, and the fibula on the outer side of the leg, which forms the outer wall of the ankle. Apply well-padded splints on both sides of leg and foot, extending from just below buttock and groin to below heel. Keep foot pointing upward. Check frequently to make sure circulation to lower leg and foot is not cut off. If splints are not available, place blanket or towels between legs and tie legs together.

ANKLE AND FOOT FRACTURE: Remove shoe and sock quickly, since swelling may be rapid. Cut off shoe and sock if necessary rather than cause further injury by pulling off. If there is an open wound, apply bulky sterile dressings if possible. Apply blanket or small pillow as a splint from several inches above the ankle to beyond the toes. Bandage in place snugly, with one tie running under the foot, another about the ankle, and the third above the second. Leave toes exposed to check circulation. Keep foot on pillow higher than knee.

PELVIC FRACTURE: The pelvis—a basin-shaped bony structure extending outward from the base of the spine and curving toward the front of the body—provides a connection between spine and legs. It also protects many important organs and blood vessels lying in the lower part of the abdomen. Because these organs and vessels may be seriously damaged by broken bone ends, a pelvic fracture is a grave injury, requiring very careful handling.

A symptom of fracture may be severe pain in the pelvic region while standing or walking; the pain may diminish or disappear while lying down. If there has been damage to organs or blood vessels, there may be difficulty in urinating or blood may appear in the urine.

If you're not certain but have any reason to suspect a fracture after an injury to the pelvic region, treat as a fracture.

Combat shock, which may be severe (see p. 14). Bandage knees and ankles together. Keep the victim lying down. He will probably be most comfortable on his back with knees straight, but let him keep his knees bent if he wishes. If he must be moved to receive medical aid, transport on back on rigid stretcher or board.

RIB FRACTURE: There is usually pain at the point of the break. Breathing is shallow since taking a deep breath or coughing increases pain. The point of fracture sometimes can be felt by running fingers gently along the rib. If the lung has been damaged by a broken rib, frothy or bright red blood may be coughed up.

If the broken rib has penetrated the skin and air is blowing in and out of the wound or just sucking into it, apply an airtight dressing. The dressing should be held firmly in place with adhesive tape and your hand. The important thing is to keep air from getting into the wound, since it will collapse the lung. Get the victim to lie quietly. If he must be moved to a doctor, move him lying down.

If the chest is not punctured, bandage firmly to restrict rib motion. To do so, first loosely tie a triangular bandage or other broad bandage around the body at chest level so the knot will be on the side opposite the break. Put a folded cloth under the knot. As the victim breathes out, tighten the bandage and tie snugly, but not so tight as to restrict breathing too much. Repeat with two or more bandages in the same way so they overlap slightly and cover the site of the fracture and adjacent areas.

NOSE FRACTURE: Look for pain and tenderness in and about the nose, swelling and discoloration, possibly a change in the usual shape of the nose. If there is bleeding, hold the lower end of the nose between thumb and index finger and firmly press the sides of the nose against the middle partition (septum) for four or five minutes. Release pressure gradually. Apply cold cloths over the nose. Have the victim sit up, hold head back slightly, and breathe through the mouth. Do not splint. If there is a wound on the nose, apply a compress or protective dressing and fix in place with adhesive tape or bandage. Get to a doctor as soon as possible.

JAW FRACTURE: Look for pain on movement and inability to close the jaw properly. Teeth do not line up correctly. There is difficulty in speaking, drinking, swallowing. Raise the jaw gently with the palm of your hand to bring lower and upper teeth together. Put a bandage under the chin and tie the ends over the top of the head to support the jaw. Remove the bandage immediately if the victim starts to vomit. Support the jaw with your hand. Rebandage when vomiting stops. If medical help is not available for several days, nourishment can be taken through a straw.

NECK OR BACK FRACTURE: If the victim is not readily able to open and close his fingers or if there is numbness or tingling around his shoulders, the neck may be broken. If his fingers work but he cannot move his feet or toes, or if he has tingling or numbness in the legs or pain when he tries to move the back or neck, his back may be broken. If the victim is unconscious and you suspect spinal injury, treat as if the neck were fractured.

Loosen clothing around neck and waist. Cover with blankets. Don't allow victim to move his head. Don't lift his head even to give him water. Any movement may cause paralysis. Watch his breathing and be ready to start resuscitation if necessary (p. 40).

Get a doctor or ambulance. The victim should not be moved unless there is no chance of getting medical help at the scene. If a move must be made, it must be done with *extreme caution*. A twist or bend of broken neck or spine can paralyze or kill. Take extreme care to avoid moving the neck or spine while loading the victim onto a rigid stretcher or board. Pad the head well at the sides to prevent motion. Tie hands across chest and tie head and body rigidly to the board. Pad under the neck.

SKULL FRACTURE: Chief reason for concern in skull fractures is not so much the bone itself as the tissues beneath it. Brain injury or concussion can occur whether there has been an actual fracture or not.

Look for a bump or cut at the site of injury. The victim

may be unconscious, or dazed and mentally confused. There may be bleeding or drainage of clear watery fluid from ears, mouth, nose. Pupils of the eyes may be different in size.

Keep the victim lying down. Prop up his head and shoulders if his face is either normal in color or flushed. Lower his head slightly if his face is pale. If a move is necessary, move the victim in lying-down position. Apply sterile gauze and bandage to an open scalp wound. Get a doctor as soon as possible but don't leave the victim alone. Keep alert. Be ready, if the victim should start choking on blood, to lower his head and turn it carefully to the side to drain the mouth. Wipe out the blood from the mouth with a clean handkerchief if necessary.

Dislocations

In a dislocation, the end of a bone is displaced from its normal position in a joint. The surrounding ligaments may suffer some injury. A dislocation may result from a fall, blow against a joint, sudden twisting of the joint, or sudden muscle contraction. Most often affected are fingers, thumb, shoulder, or elbow.

Symptoms may include swelling, obvious deformity, pain upon motion, tenderness to touch, discoloration.

Putting a serious dislocation back into place (i.e., "reducing" it) is a physician's job. Unless properly relocated and cared for, there may be repeated dislocation and disability. All dislocations should be handled in much the same way as fractures.

Keep the dislocated part quiet. Don't try to reduce it. Splint and immobilize the joint in the dislocated position. Apply cold compresses. Seek medical attention promptly.

Support a dislocated elbow or shoulder in a loose sling so it is kept immobilized during transport. If a hip is dislocated, move the victim on a wide board or stretcher made rigid. Use a pad of blankets or clothing large enough to support the leg on the injured side in the position the victim holds it.

Sometimes, in the case of a dislocated finger, when medical attention will be long delayed, gentle traction may be tried. Pull cautiously—very cautiously—on the finger to try to bring the bone into place. If unsuccessful, do not persist. And do not attempt this on a dislocated thumb, since there are more difficulties in the way and more risk of added injury.

One of the most common ski injuries is thumb dislocation. It results from grasping the top of the pole and ski strap between thumb and index finger. The slightest fall puts tremendous twisting force on the base of the thumb, pushing it out of its socket. To avoid this injury, either put your hand downward through the loop of the strap and grasp only the pole, with the loop lying loosely around the wrist—or, better still, use a strapless pole or a strap that detaches automatically from the pole under pressure.

Sprains

Sprains, as noted previously, are injuries to soft tissues surrounding joints, with stretching and sometimes tearing or partial tearing of ligaments, muscles, tendons, and blood vessels. Ankles, fingers, wrists, and knees are most commonly affected.

Symptoms include swelling, tenderness, pain or

motion, and sometimes discoloration of skin over a large area because of rupture of small blood vessels.

It is often difficult even for a physician to tell a sprain from a fracture without an x-ray. If the sprain seems severe, or if you have any reason to suspect a fracture, splint the part and treat as you would a fracture.

Otherwise, rest and elevate the injured part. If ankle or knee is affected, there should be no walking. Loosen or remove shoes. Swelling, because it can cut off circulation, may sometimes cause more trouble than the original sprain. To minimize swelling, elevate the leg and apply cold compresses. Cold helps contract blood vessels, minimize leakage of blood, tends to reduce swelling and pain. For wrist sprain, put the arm in a sling adjusted so the fingers are about four inches higher than the elbow. For elbow sprain, also put the arm in a sling. Apply cold compresses.

In mild sprains, keep the injured part immobilized and raised for at least 24 hours, continuing the cold applications.

If swelling and pain persist, get medical help.

Strains

Strains are muscle injuries due to overexertion, with muscle fibers stretched, sometimes partially torn. While strains can occur in any muscle, most frequent are those of back muscles, usually caused by lifting.

Symptoms include sharp pain or cramp at the time of injury; stiffness and pain on movement, which may increase within a few hours; and some swelling of the affected muscle.

Have the victim rest the injured area, sitting or lying

quietly in a comfortable position. Apply hot compresses. Massage gently—in the direction of the heart, to stimulate blood flow in that direction. Gentle massage may help lessen stiffness. For a strained back, a bed board under the mattress helps by providing firm support.

Headaches

It would be difficult to conceive of a more unlikely cause of puzzling headaches than bedcovers—more accurately, sleeping with bedcovers over the head. Yet such headaches, aptly named "turtle" headaches, have been reported in a series of patients—and until identified for what they are they can be quite mysterious, awakening victims from sleep during the night or striking upon arising in the morning, generalized, the whole head hurting. The cure is simple enough: Give up the covers-over-the-head habit that apparently causes headache by depriving the brain of adequate oxygen.

Headaches, of course, can accompany many diseases along with other symptoms, such as fever, muscle aches and pains in flu.

But headache without any other associated symptoms is most commonly of the tension or muscle contraction type in which, usually as the result of emotional or other stress but sometimes because of strained posture (as in driving in a rainstorm, for example), neck, and scalp, and even jaw muscles may go into spasm. For such headaches, aspirin is often helpful, especially if coupled with other measures such as massage or heat applied to the back of the neck and resting with eyes closed and the head supported.

Recently, for some sufferers with often-repeated tension headaches, biofeedback has been found useful. If you belong in this category, you may want to try feedback, which essentially is a method of relaxation now being offered in many hospital headache clinics. Typically, electrodes are placed on the forehead (a totally painless procedure) to record muscle tension. With tension level high, the biofeedback equipment may emit rapid beeps. As tension is reduced, the beeps come more slowly. And as you learn—in some fashion difficult to explain—to make the beeps slow down, with the aid of the biofeedback equipment, you note what you are doing to achieve the feat and then may be able to reproduce it without the equipment, as a means of stopping a headache before it has time to really get started.

MIGRAINE: Many of what are called migraine headaches are really severe tension headaches and would better be treated that way. True migraine headaches often are preceded by visual disturbances such as "seeing stars" and accompanied by nausea. They affect one side of the head, although the side may vary from one attack to another. Migraine headaches involve constriction and relaxation of blood vessels in the head. Drugs that affect blood vessels, such as Cafergot, may help migraine but not tension headaches.

If you're a migraine victim, you may not have been getting adequate relief from medications such as Cafergot. The problem may lie with taking medication when nausea is already present; when nausea is present, the stomach often absorbs medication poorly. One maneuver you may find helpful in determining whether a migraine or another kind of headache is coming is to sit down and place your head between your knees. If the head throbs, a migraine episode is very probably on its way, and medication for it should be taken immediately.

Is diet involved in migraine? Recent research does suggest that certain foods can, in the migraine-prone, have an effect on blood vessels that may trigger attacks. They include red wines and champagne, aged or strong cheese (particularly cheddar), pickled herring, chicken livers, pods of broad beans, and canned figs. Their avoidance may be helpful.

For some people, cured meats, including frankfurters, bacon, ham, and salami, may have adverse effects, and a trial of avoiding them may be worthwhile. Monosodium glutamate, a salt used to enhance the flavor of foods, may in large amounts trigger migraine, and excesses should be avoided.

Recently, too, biofeedback has been used with reported success to reduce the frequency and intensity of migraine headaches. There has also been some success for people unresponsive to usual migraine medications with propranolol, a drug often used for heart patients, and, in other cases, with amitriptyline, an antidepressant drug often used for mental depression.

OTHER HEADACHES: Nitrites are chemical compounds that may be used as preservatives in cured meats, and at least one recent study indicates that in some people sensitive to nitrites they may be responsible for otherwise mysterious headaches—moderately severe, nonthrobbing, usually lasting several hours and sometimes accompanied by facial flushing. If you happen to be sensitive to nitrites, such headaches may occur within half an hour after eating such cured meat products as frankfurters, bacon, salami, and ham, which contain the compounds.

CAFFEINISM—excessive intake of caffeine in the form of coffee, tea, cola drinks, and even medications that contain caffeine— has been linked with some cases of what appear to be severe, recurrent tension headaches. If you're a frequent headache sufferer and also a heavy partaker of caffeine, you may want to try minimizing your caffeine intake to see if that helps.

Persistent headaches that do not respond to any of the measures you can try at home should have medical attention—preferably the kind of expert attention you may get from a physician or clinic specializing in headache diagnosis and treatment. Chances are, if you inquire, you can find such a physician or clinic not too far from you.

Head Injuries

No injury to the head, however seemingly slight or trivial, should be ignored.

It may or may not be serious.

If you observe certain guidelines, you can avoid needless anxiety, on the one hand, and neglect of something serious, on the other.

Typically, in a *minor* head injury, there may be a quickly developing bump, some initial stunning, but no loss of consciousness. Especially in a child, there may even be an episode of vomiting or two in the first few hours, which then stops. Not long afterward, all is well except perhaps the swollen bump, which will disappear in due course.

WHAT TO DO FOR MINOR INJURY: Apply ice as soon as possible to minimize the size of the swelling. If there is a bleeding scalp wound—and scalp wounds tend to bleed profusely—raise the victim's head and shoulders to control the bleeding. Apply a sterile dressing snugly on the wound, and when bleeding is under control, bandage the dressing to hold it in place.

WHAT TO DO FOR MORE SEVERE INJURY: In a more severe injury, there may be immediate or delayed indications.

Get medial help without delay if a clear or blood-tinged fluid drains from the nose and ear; it may indicate a skull fracture. Get medical help, too, in case of unconsciousness.

Until medical help is available, keep the victim lying down. Lying quietly helps to lessen the possibility or extent of hemorrhage within the skull.

If the victim is unconscious or having difficulty breathing, turn his head gently to the side to allow blood or mucus to drain from the corner of the mouth.

A valuable trick if you are alone with a person who has a scalp laceration: Use the victim's hair as a suture (stitch). Take a few hairs on each side of the cut and tie them to each other, so the edges of the wound are pulled together, closing it and controlling the bleeding. Tie three knots in each set of hair strands. Repeat with other strands until the wound is closed. The knots may tend to pull apart if the hair is oily; if you have collodion available, touch some to the knots and hold until the collodion sticks. Then apply a sterile dressing.

Note: Even in the absence of potentially serious indications such as fluid draining from the nose and ear or unconsciousness, anyone who has had more than a very mild head injury should restrict activity for 24 hours and not be left alone.

And a watch should be kept for any of the following signs, which may indicate possible brain damage:

• Variable consciousness: Periods of drowsiness interspersed with alertness can indicate increasing pressure on the brain.

• The pupils of the eyes—the small black circles inside the colored rings in the center of the eyes—should be the same size in both eyes and should contract in size when a light is shined into the eyes. If they are unequal in size and fail to contract when exposed to light, there may be increased brain pressure and urgent need for medical help.

• Irrational or unusual behavior, including unusual restlessness, may be a warning.

• Severe, recurrent, and often forceful vomiting calls for medical help.

• Irregular, slow, and deep breathing may indicate increased brain pressure and need for medical attention.

• Arm or leg muscle weakness, drooping of an eye or one side of the mouth, or tingling, numbness or paralysis in one arm or leg may indicate brain damage and need for medical help.

• A change of vision, particularly blurring or double vision, if it persists, calls for medical attention.

• Persistent or severe headache may mean serious injury—but note that after any head injury headache is not unusual. An ordinary headache, however, usually tends to gradually decrease rather than intensify. Apply an ice pack or cold wet towel and use aspirin if needed but avoid anything stronger—and if these measures do nothing for the headache, medical help is probably needed.

Note: Sometimes, days or weeks after a head injury and an apparently good recovery, there may be late changes indicating trouble. Some confusion, a change in personality (often slight), and increasing somnolence may indicate a slowly increasing blood clot within the skull (subdural hematoma) which is compressing the brain and requires medical attention.

REMEMBER:

1. Control scalp bleeding; it can be profuse.
2. Careful observation is necessary to recognize complications early.
3. Clear or blood-tinged fluid from nose or ear may indicate a skull fracture.

Influenza (Flu)

A severe but usually relatively brief respiratory infection, influenza is caused by three groups of viruses, called A (which includes Asian flu), B, and C. Each group has variant viruses but all produce similar symptoms that vary only in intensity.

Spread by droplets from sneezes and coughs, influenza is highly contagious, with an incubation period of about 48 hours before symptoms appear.

The first symptoms, which often develop suddenly, are chilliness and fever up to 102° or 103°F. Other early symptoms include prostration and generalized aches and pains, which are most pronounced in the back and legs. Headache is common and is often accompanied by sensitivity to light. Respiratory symptoms—sore throat, burning below the breastbone, nonproductive cough, and sometimes nasal discharge—may be mild at first but later may become more pronounced.

Usually, after two or three days, symptoms begin to

subside rapidly and fever is over (but sometimes fever may last as long as five days without complications). Fatigue, weakness, and excessive sweating may persist for several days or sometimes several weeks after other symptoms are gone.

WHAT TO DO: During the stage of acute symptoms and for 24 to 48 hours after temperature drops to normal, adequate rest—preferably bed rest—and avoidance of exertion are indicated.

For fever and discomfort, one or two 5-grain tablets of aspirin* every four hours can be taken. If nasal obstruction is severe, one or two drops of 0.25 percent phenylephrine (as in Neo-Synephrine, for example) instilled into the nose often help. Excessive use of the drops, however, should be avoided since that may cause a rebound reaction and increased stuffiness. Warm salt-water gargles are helpful for sore throat. Steam inhalation is often very useful in relieving respiratory symptoms.

Special note: There is a drug, amantadine hydrochloride, which your physician may prescribe for influenza. It is often used for shaking palsy (parkinsonism), but it has also been found to have some usefulness for influenza. Amantadine appears to be antiviral in this sense: it has no direct effect on flu viruses themselves but rather acts to decrease their penetration into body cells where they can multiply.

When there is an epidemic of flu of severe type, the physician may prescribe amantadine early in the disease when it may sometimes considerably alleviate symptoms.

---

*NOTE: *Aspirin must not be given to children since it can result in Reye's Syndrome, a life-threatening condition.*

The drug also can be prescribed for preventive purposes for family members and others in close contact with the sick one and, generally, for people at high risk because of age or chronic health problems.

Leg Cramps

Almost everyone has experienced a painful muscle cramp. When a muscle, especially one that has had relatively little use, is exercised too violently, it may react by contracting and failing to relax, producing a painful cramp.

WHAT TO DO: Heat, particularly from warm baths, is helpful, and two aspirin tablets every four hours also will be useful in relieving discomfort.

People who exercise vigorously, especially in hot weather, may develop leg cramps through loss of sodium and potassium in perspiration. The two elements are needed for efficient nervous system functioning, and with their excessive loss, faulty nerve function may overstimulate muscles, causing violent contraction and cramps. Usually, this can be avoided with well-balanced meals that include foods rich in sodium and potassium and other important substances. Such foods include chicken, eggs, liver, milk, citrus fruits, bananas, and dark-green leafy vegetables. For an attack, heat may help; so, too, stretching the muscle out as much as you can while massaging above the aching area to encourage blood flow into it.

If you tend to get leg cramps fairly often with strenuous activity, try making it a practice to do a few minutes of easy warm-up exercises beforehand and some easy cool-down exercises afterward.

Night Leg Cramps

Cramps of leg and foot muscles that awaken one from sleep constitute a common complaint. The attacks may be relatively mild and infrequent or may occur several times a night, forcing you to get out of bed, walk about, rub the muscles, and try anything to get relief.

The cause is not always clear but usually has nothing to do with blood circulation. When poor circulation causes leg discomfort, it does so with effort rather than at rest.

WHAT TO DO: If you are taking a diuretic drug ("water pill"), that may possibly be involved because it leads to excretion of potassium, and you may benefit by increasing your intake of potassium-rich foods such as citrus fruits and bananas. Sometimes, potassium loss with a diuretic may require use of a prescribed potassium preparation.

Otherwise, many measures have been used, with varying success, to try to prevent nightly leg cramps. Some people who notice that their attacks happen more often when their feet are cool benefit by wearing socks to bed. Some benefit from elevating the legs with a pillow, which may indicate that, at least for them, pooling of blood in the legs may be a factor; the leg elevation helps return of blood from legs to heart. For some people, quinine taken at bedtime is useful.

Vitamin E has recently been reported to be effective in many cases. It is taken in the form of *d*-alpha-tocopherol acetate or succinate. Dosages used have ranged from 400 international units once a day to four times a day, although people with high blood pressure or heart problems and those with diabetes taking insulin should start

with much smaller doses; and it would be wise for them
to consult a physician first. Because inorganic iron com-
bines with and inactivates vitamin E, vitamin preparations containing iron, and white bread or cereals fortified
with iron, should be avoided.

Muscle and Joint Pain, Tenderness, Stiffness (Fibromyositis)

Usually caused by injury, strain, exposure to damp or
cold, and occasionally by infection, fibromyositis is an
inflammation of muscle tissue and the connective tissue
of joints and muscles.

It produces pain, often sudden in onset, which is
aggravated by movement. Tenderness and stiffness also
develop. Most often affected are the low back, shoulders,
chest, and thighs.

WHAT TO DO: Fibromyositis may disappear spontaneously in a few days or weeks but sometimes may become
chronic or reappear at intervals.

Simple home measures often can provide relief: rest,
local applications of heat, gentle massage, and two aspirin or acetaminophen tablets every three or four hours.

In severe, persistent, or recurrent cases, the problem
may lie with very sensitive little areas in muscles called
trigger points. Aptly named, trigger points—like gun trig-
gers—can fire off pain to another place, a target area.

A trigger point in the shoulder may shoot pain to neck
and shoulder that may seem to be due to arthritis of the
neck area of the spine—or it can cause tingling sensations
in the neck and forearm, or headaches with the pain
distributed to the top of the skull. A trigger point in the
low back area can cause low back and sometimes sciatica-

like pain shooting down the leg.

A trigger point may result from excessive exercise, a sudden twist, strain or sprain, even sleeping in poor position. Poor posture may be accountable. And fatigue, chilling, and anxiety may contribute.

Once the possibility of a trigger point is considered, you may be able to find it at home, or your physician can find it—and, in any case, if a trigger point is the problem, you will need medical help.

When a fingertip is applied firmly to a trigger point, sudden intensification of the typical pain makes the diagnosis obvious. But it make take systematic exploration to find the trigger point because it may be at a distance from the painful area.

Once the point is found, the physician can inject a small amount of a local anesthetic, such as Novocain, Xylocaine, or Carbocaine, directly into the area. Sometimes, a cortisonelike drug may be injected along with the anesthetic.

Discomfort intensifies during the injection, but pain and tenderness usually disappear within a few minutes. In some cases, a single injection may be enough; in chronic cases, a series of injections given every four to seven days may be needed for long-lasting relief.

Pneumonia

Pneumonia, an infection of the lungs, can be caused by various bacteria and viruses and by oily material and other foreign matter that get into the lungs.

Bacterial Pneumonia

This is the most common type. It is infectious and can

be spread from person to person, usually through the air.

The lungs are divided into five lobes. If one or more lobes are affected, the infection is called *lobar pneumonia*; infection of both lungs is called *double* or *bilateral pneumonia*. *Bronchopneumonia* refers to pneumonia that is localized mainly in or around the bronchial tubes; it is usually but not always milder than lobar pneumonia.

Pneumonia often begins as, or may be preceded by, a respiratory infection such as the common cold. When the lungs become involved, the disease is not difficult to identify.

There may be a sudden, shaking chill. High fever follows. Other cardinal symptoms include sharp chest pains, cough, and blood-streaked or rusty brown sputum.

WHAT TO DO: Anyone with these symptoms should get into bed and remain there, and a physician should be called immediately.

Pneumonia is an emergency disease. Although there has been some tendency since the advent of antibiotics to dismiss the disease as no longer important, it is potentially dangerous and requires prompt and adequate treatment.

A suitable antibiotic must be started at once, even while a phlegm or smear sample is sent to a laboratory. Once the particular bacterium is identified by the laboratory, the physician may change to a still better antibiotic for that organism.

Complete bed rest is required. The patient should be isolated, with few or no visitors, and masks should be worn if possible.

Plenty of liquids should be taken, and a suitable diet will be ordered by the physician. A tight ·chest binder against which the patient can cough may be helpful.

The outlook for pneumonia when antibiotic treatment is instituted promptly is excellent. Chances for recovery are about 95 out of 100.

PREVENTION: Good general health is an important protective factor; when the body is weakened, resistance to pneumonia organisms is lowered.

New vaccines against pneumonia are being developed. One, for example, now available to immunize against pneumococcal pneumonia, which is the most common bacterial form, is 90 percent effective and may be especially valuable for people in older age groups and those with chronic diseases such as diabetes and heart, liver and kidney disease, who may be particularly susceptible.

Legionnaire's Disease

In the summer of 1976, a mysterious epidemic of severe pneumonialike disease struck 180 persons in Philadelphia, most of whom were attending an American Legion convention. There were 29 fatalities.

The disease was characterized by fever, cough, and chest x-ray evidence of pneumonia. It took intensive investigation before a particular organism—a Gram-negative bacterium—could be not only isolated from lung tissue of disease victims but also established as the causative agent.

Much remains to be learned about the disease. Since the Philadelphia outbreak, other cases have been reported. What the prevalence may be throughout the country is not yet known.

Recently, too, researchers have been finding that there are at least two separate forms of Legionnaire's disease. Although both are caused by the same bacterium, a second form is not potentially fatal. It is more influenzalike, with the victim experiencing headache, fever, and muscle ache.

Meanwhile, progress has been made in identifying and treating the disease, including the potentially fatal form.

Tests to confirm the presence of the disease, originally developed by the National Center for Disease Control in Atlanta, now can be carried out by almost all state laboratories and many private laboratories. Other tests also are being developed.

The tests are vital. Legionnaire's disease does not respond to all antibiotics. Penicillin, for example, seems useless. Good results, however, have been achieved with certain other antibiotics—erythromycin, in particular. There have also been reports of improvement with the antibiotics chloramphenicol and tetracycline.

WHAT TO DO: Any pneumonia that produces severe symptoms is, as already noted, an emergency disease.

Along with fever, breathing difficulty, cough, and blood in the sputum, Legionnaire's disease may produce other symptoms which do not necessarily distinguish it from other forms of pneumonia: muscle pains, severe headache, vomiting, diarrhea, delirium.

Get into bed; get a physician. Antibiotic treatment may be started immediately, and the particular antibiotic may be changed according to what laboratory tests indicate.

Like other pneumonias, so with Legionnaire's dis-

ease: chances for successful recovery are greatly
improved by prompt and suitable care.

Atypical (Viral) Pneumonia

This type of pneumonia differs somewhat from bacterial pneumonias. Although it is often called viral or
virus pneumonia, it may be caused more often by organisms called *Mycoplasma*, which are a kind of bacteria,
rather than by viruses.

The onset is gradual. There are mild cases in which
symptoms are much like those of the common cold. In
other cases, there may be mild chills and fever. Cough is
common. Severe headache, muscle aches, and loss of
appetite may be present.

WHAT TO DO: A physician should be called. Atypical
pneumonia, if caused by *Mycoplasma* bacteria, usually
responds well to the antibiotic tetracycline.

Even without specific medication, the disease tends to
be self-limiting. Bed rest is important. Codeine or
another agent may be needed for cough. Steam inhalation is useful.

Rest for a few days after fever is gone may help to
avoid extended fatigue and weakness.

Aspiration Pneumonia

Aspiration, medically, means the act of breathing or
drawing in. An aspiration pneumonia is one caused by
foreign matter drawn into the lungs.

Aspiration pneumonia may follow anesthesia, alco-
holic intoxication, convulsive disorders, and disturbances of consciousness associated with vomiting which
may permit some of the vomitus to be drawn into the

lungs. It may sometimes follow the improper administration of oily nose drops, especially in children and older people. Oily noise drops should be administered carefully, with the patient on his back, head tilted far back and turned to the side.

If enough foreign matter reaches the lungs, infection can occur. Symptoms may include fever, chest pains, cough, and shortness of breath.

WHAT TO DO: Prompt medical help is needed. A tube may be used to remove as much as possible of the foreign material. Oxygen may be administered. If acid stomach contents have gotten into the lungs, a cortisonelike drug may be administered by injection. A suitable antibiotic can be used.

In a recent medical report, a nurse noted using the Heimlich maneuver to expel vomitus that has been aspirated into the lungs of a patient.

Poison Ivy, Poison Oak

Contact with this and other *Rhus* (sumac family) plants at any season can produce an allergic skin reaction. The reaction may also develop through indirect contact via pets, contaminated clothing, or smoke from burning plants. It produces, after 12 to 48 hours, an itching rash which may persist for as long as two weeks.

WHAT TO DO: The irritating substance is the oily sap in leaves, flowers, fruit, stem, bark, and roots. Prompt washing of the skin with yellow laundry soap after exposure often helps prevent a reaction.

When only a few small blisters are present, warm water compressed applied for brief internals may provide some relief. Alternatively, calamine lotion or a compress soaked in dilute Burow's solution (1 pint to 15 pints of cool water) may be applied.

If itching is too severe to be tolerated despite home measures, if there are large blisters, severe inflammation, or fever, or if the face or genital area is severely affected, seeing a physician is advisable. A cream containing a cortisonelike agent to be applied several times a day or a cortisonelike drug to be taken by mouth may be prescribed.

Rashes

Rashes accompany many diseases, usually along with other symptoms. These are some of the more common rash-producing illnesses, with the types of rashes they produce and other accompanying symptoms:

Measles: Pink spots, each about one-fourth inch in diameter, often start at the hairline and behind the ears and spread downward to cover the body in about 36 hours, with the spots separate at first but some, later, running together to give a blotchy look, fading after three or four days; with running nose, cough, slight fever, pains in head and back, reddened eyes.

German measles: The rash is much like that of measles but the spots do not usually coalesce; they fade after two or three days; with slight cold, sore throat.

Roseola: A pinkish rash appears after three or four days of fever, usually just as the fever is beginning to decline, and lasts a few days.

Biography of
Dr. Henry J. Heimlich

Dr. Henry J. Heimlich, President, The Heimlich Institute, has been credited with saving more lives than any other living American. Over 20,000 lives have been saved by the HEIMLICH MANEUVER in the U.S. alone. Former Surgeon General C. Everett Koop declared:

"The best rescue technique in any choking situation is the Heimlich Maneuver. I urge the American Red Cross, The American Heart Association, and all those who teach first aid to teach only the Heimlich Maneuver."

A partial list of Dr. Heimlich's other accomplishments are:

CANCER: The Heimlich Institute is currently preparing to treat otherwise incurable cancer patients with Dr. Heimlich's malariatherapy technique.

CYSTIC FIBROSIS & EMPHYSEMA: The Heimlich Micro Trach (HMT) is used to treat children with cystic fibrosis to expel mucus, promoting health and prevention of infection. It also allows bedridden patients to become mobile, and return to work and social activities with the use of a small portable oxygen container.

STROKE: He has devised methods to help victims of stroke to swallow again through a procedure called "Relearning the Swallowing Process."

HEIMLICH OPERATION: The Heimlich Operation for constructing a new esophagus, devised in the 1950s, was the first successful replacement in history of an internal organ and is now used in operating rooms throughout the world.

CHEST VALVE: The Heimlich Valve for Chest Drainage is credited with saving hundreds of lives in the Vietnam

War and now is used extensively in military and civilian medicine.

Educated at Cornell University and Cornell Medical College, Dr. Heimlich was a surgical resident at Mt. Sinai and Bellevue Hospitals in New York City. During World War II he served as a surgeon in the United States Naval Group China (classified as voluntary extrahazardous overseas duty) involving two years in China behind Japanese lines.

He has received numerous awards and commendations including being enshrined in the Engineering and Science Hall of Fame in 1984, Albert Lasker Public Service Award in 1984, and the American Academy Achievement Golden Plate Award in 1985.